# WHIPPING HIDDEN ALLERGIES

by

## Harris W. Hosen, M.D.

NON FICTITIOUS PRESS

Cover art by *Texas Highways Magazine*

Library of Congress Card Catalog No. 93-087091 Harris W.
        Hosen, M.D.        192pp
            Whipping Hidden Allergies
    1. Allergies.


ISBN # 0-9622762-3-5  Hard cover
ISBN # 0-9622762-2-7  Soft cover

Printed in the United States of America

*The author, agent and publisher offer this book as a helpful guideline to the lay reader. Final diagnosis and treatment should always be under the direction and care of qualified and licensed medical personnel in direct contact with the patient.*

*All names mentioned in the case studies are fictitious.*

*Dedicated to my family*

# TABLE OF CONTENTS

# ABOUT THE AUTHOR

Harris Hosen, MD, graduated from medical school at Tulane University in 1931 and took his residency in Pediatrics at Touro Infirmary in New Orleans. This was followed by a year on the pediatric faculty at Louisiana State University Medical School. Dr. Hosen then spent a preceptorship with a leading allergist, Dr. Bernard Efron, in New Orleans.

For 30 years, Dr. Hosen practiced pediatrics and allergy in Port Arthur, Texas. When he went into provocative allergy testing 20 years ago, it proved to be such an efficient method of treating patients that he dropped pediatrics entirely and isolated himself to allergy alone.

Dr. Hosen is a Fellow in the American College of Allergy, the Society of Clinical Ecology, and the American Association of Allergy and Immunology. He is a recipient of the Jonathan Forman Gold Medal Award given by the Ecology Society in 1981 for his contributions toward cures for allergy. He published a book for the allergy profession in 1978 entitled, *Clinical Allergy Based On Provocative Testing.*

Dr. Hosen has been a guest speaker at two international allergy symposiums, in England and Holland. In addition, he has spoken on the programs of allergy societies and is the author of numerous publications in allergy journals.

# OVERVIEW

The purpose of this work is to acquaint the public with a departure from the traditional methods of allergy identification and to introduce a new type of investigation. A true and accurate determination of whether an allergy is or is not responsible for specific symptoms can be simple, accurate, and inexpensive. My method of diagnosis is based upon provccative tests rather than traditional skin tests. Provocative tests have shown exceptional reliability over the past 20 years, particularly when compared with the results of the traditional methods I had personally used during the previous 30 years.

The use of skin tests has a reliability factor of approximately 30 per cent, which I have proved by special investigations. Provocative testing, as used in this book, refers to the reproduction of the patient's symptoms. The tests I devised have an accuracy of 90 per cent. This is a far cry from the 30 per cent using traditional methods. Further, my technique is safe and dependable.

From the physician/patient point of view, each patient is told in writing that, if he is allergic to inhalants with or without foods, within three to six months of treatment he must be cured or near cured of all symptoms. If foods alone are the culprit, a cure is complete upon elimination of the foods involved. If after six months such results are not achieved, a new investigation is made without charge to the patient.

On several patients, the missing link to a cure or near cure was found to be the *sulfite chemical so* prevalent in a number of foods and drinks. This condition can be isolated by provocative testing in the medical office. The patient is given a large dose of the *sulfite chemical* contained in two capsules on an empty stomach. If allergic, a reaction will occur within 30 minutes. Such reactions are easily controlled within minutes. I exhibited this approach to curing allergies during 1985 at the convention of the American College of Allergists and at the American Association of Allergy and Immunology demonstrated a specific treatment for this sensitivity that brings about a clinical cure within six months.

Patients treated by traditional methods are told that it takes up to three years of desensitizing injections to obtain relief. If the patient does not get relief, many traditional allergists insist if the condition does not get worse then the patient should consider the situation as *good results,* as allergy is progressive and *treatment* has stopped the progress of the disease. By and large, patients accept this and take injections for years, often relying on drugstore medications for relief.

Traditional allergists have just begun to acknowledge the important place of foods in clinical allergy! For years, I have stressed that foods are involved in 75 per cent of the allergic patients. This book presents proof of exactly that.

# 1

## *INTRODUCTION*

The doctor gives you a complicated series of skin tests, says you have allergies, then tells you that three to five years of *his shots* should help you feel better. Sound familiar?

The diagnosis and treatment plan is a middle of the road approach. After all, you have been bothered by a variety of aches and pains most of your life. So you reason that it ought to take three to five years to feel better, and it ought to be expensive.

Hogwash!

Testing for allergies can be simple, inexpensive, and accurate. With proper treatment, an allergy sufferer should be significantly better, if not cured, in three to five months! Not years, months!

The staggering difference between months and years for relief is the difference between my methods of determining the cause of an allergy and other methods traditionally used by doctors. If you don't know the exact cause of the allergy, you cannot eliminate it. You can treat the symptoms, but you cannot solve the problem.

To solve the problem, the allergy sufferer must avoid, if possible, the allergens which are the substances that cause the allergic reaction. If you are allergic to feathers, relief could be as

1

simple as trading your goosefeather pillow for a cotton headrest. If you cannot avoid the irritating substances such as house dust or dander from the family dog, you may require desensitizing injections for relief.

By definition, an allergy is being hypersensitive (overly sensitive) to some *plant, animal, insect, chemical, or food. If* you remove the offending material or become less sensitive to it, your symptoms will go away.

However, if the allergy sufferer does not receive satisfactory relief in three to five months, the cause of the allergy was incorrectly identified, or something else, either missed during testing or not included in the testing process, is making life miserable for the individual. In such cases, the allergy sufferer needs to be retested to properly identify the cause of the problem. The person does not need years of costly treatment that will only work by luck or accident.

One allergist, for example, reported in a national journal that after treating 350 cases of bronchial asthma, he had 15 per cent failures, 15 per cent cures, and 70 per cent *good results,* but it took three to five years of treatment to attain those *good results.* The fact is, in three to five years, patients can get better by chance, by adapting or getting used to whatever causes their allergies, or by plain outgrowing such allergies. *Good results,* indeed!

Allergy accounts for more illness than many people realize. People are familiar with things that cause common allergies such as plant pollen (hay fever), house dust, pets, molds, and insects. But the fact is that 70 per cent of allergy patients are allergic to one or more foods. In fact, most people are allergic to something, but their allergies do not bother them enough to require treatment.

The most common allergy symptoms include sneezing, coughing, nasal congestion, red and watery eyes, headaches, shortness of breath, and wheezing. Allergies can also involve the gastrointestinal tract (stomach and intestines), the central nervous system, urinary system, muscles, joints, and skin. Allergy is a great imitator, and allergic reactions in these areas of the body can look like any disease known to man. THAT IS WHY ANY CHRONIC CONDITION SHOULD BE CONSIDERED ALLERGIC UNTIL PROVEN OTHERWISE. If you have a pain or ailment that does not go away, look for an allergy and look beyond your nose. Nasal congestion and breathing difficulties are tip-offs that allergies are involved, but those same symptoms are commonly present as secondary or accompanying symptoms to many other allergic reactions.

If you are allergic to the chemicals the local drive-in restaurant uses to keep the salads looking fresh, all the hay fever allergy shots in the world will not keep your nose from running (the secondary symptoms) or cure the unexplained acne (the primary allergic reaction) you develop every time you eat there. However, you might find an allergist who would treat your *hay fever* with years of shots, a prescription for decongestive medication, and advice to see a dermatologist for your complexion. The ability of allergies to imitate the symptoms of other illnesses and create medical smoke screens makes them difficult to treat. In fact, most allergies go untreated because they are not recognized as allergic reactions.

Generally, when an illness is not controlled by routine medical treatment and vague symptoms continue, many doctors do not look for an allergy solution. Instead, doctors usually look for a mental one. The person with the vague, persistent complaints is labeled psychoneurotic and told *it's all in your head*. The doctor then forgets the patient, and the patient frequently wanders from doctor to doctor wondering why no one will help. These people do not die, and they often are reasonably successful at their jobs despite chronic illness. Yet, they never really feel well. These patients I call *the forgotten people*.

Many of my patients were *forgotten people.* John Monahan, a building contractor and avid swimmer in the San Antonio area, had been to many doctors and received various tests and medications before coming to see me. The pain was not in his head but in his joints, and he could not get relief. I finally hospitalized him in a controlled environment where I could monitor what he ate, drank, and breathed. After exhaustive testing, I could find no cause. But, strangely, his symptoms cleared up! He checked out of the hospital and went home. The next day he called and complained of joint pain. Had he stayed on his diets? Yes. What did he do after leaving the hospital and upon arriving at home? He drank city water and took a dip in his swimming pool. Testing confirmed that John was allergic to chlorine! The danger of a severe asthmatic attack occurring while in the swimming pool cannot be overemphasized. Potentially, it could have caused incapacitation and death by drowning. John drained his pool and switched to the bromine agent for purifying and, as well, immediately cut out drinking city water and installed a water purifying system at his home. Today, John's allergy is under control, and he is no longer *forgotten.*

Results have been poor in traditional allergy treatment since German pediatrician Baron Clemens von Pirquet first used the term allergy to describe sensitivity to tuberculin, a test for tuberculosis, in 1906. Physicians in other medical specialties tended to view allergy as the *bastard* field of medicine, more closely allied with black magic and quackery than scientific medicine.

Having practiced allergy for 50 years, I am familiar with traditional methods, having used them for 30 years. However, the methods I developed during the past 20 years for identifying allergies have proved exceptionally reliable in providing relief for the *forgotten people.*

True allergy practice means finding specific causes of the allergic condition and eliminating those causes. It does not mean playing the patient/potion guessing game arrived at by taking shots in the dark like some witch doctor hoping to get *good results*.

# 2

# *PROVOCATIVE NASAL TESTS FOR DIAGNOSIS OF INHALANT ALLERGENS: CORRELATION WITH SKIN TESTS AND CLINICAL SYMPTOMS*

The car salesman has a deal for you. Seven out of ten new cars on the sales lot do not have engines. You pick out the car you want and pay for it without looking under the hood. Sound like a good deal? Of course not, but thousands of people engage in the medical equivalent of this same kind of deal everyday by getting treatment, usually desensitizing injections or shots, that will not help them overcome their allergies.

The treatment will not help because it is often based upon skin tests that are not accurate in detecting the causes of allergies. Frequently, those tests are only 30 per cent accurate! Another way of looking at it: three out of ten people obtain some relief from their allergies via this method while seven out of ten are totally wasting their money!

By and large, doctors are not deliberately bilking patients with unnecessary treatments, but the track record of traditional tests used to identify the causes of allergies almost makes it seem that way. I have made careful studies comparing the success rates of different tests and will discuss those results later in this chapter.

For starters, what are the traditional methods of identifying the causes of allergies, and how do provocative methods differ? The common methods allergists use for identifying allergies are patient histories, diaries, scratch tests, and intradermal or injection-type tests. I have used these methods and find they do not compare with the results obtained using the provocative testing methods I have personally developed.

Some allergists stress the importance of a good patient history. To be sure, a good history is useful as a starting point in identifying an allergy's cause. Unfortunately, it is too frequently a stopping point. When a history suggests dust, mold, or pollen allergies, it cannot help to determine specifically which dusts, molds, or pollens are the culprits.

For example, your son becomes ill every year when the family brings a live Christmas tree into the house. An allergist who depends upon histories might say that he is surely allergic to tree molds. That is surely possible. He could also be allergic to the eggnog the family shares along with the ritual of decorating the tree. A history suggests things that may be factors in an allergy, but it cannot confirm the causes.

Diaries fall into the same category as histories. The allergy sufferer records his or her activities in a diary, and those activities are compared to the person's symptoms. An allergist who depends on diaries might say that Mary, for example, is allergic to something she ate for lunch on Tuesday because she started sneezing after lunch. That is surely possible. Mary may also be allergic to smoke from the cigarette a friend smoked after the meal, an incident Mary forgot to include in her diary. Again, a diary can be helpful, but it will not isolate a cause.

The two most common methods of detecting allergies, the scratch test and the intradermal or *inside the skin* test, are the chief tools traditional doctors use to identify allergies. *Scratch tests* are made with a sharp, metal tool called a *scarifier* which breaks the top layers of skin without drawing blood. The doctor or assistant then puts a drop of solution containing the material being tested (e.g., house dust) on the torn skin. The solution is rubbed in, and the spot is checked within 15 minutes for a *reaction*. The test is considered positive if a red bump similar to an insect bite appears *Intradermal tests* are made with a hypodermic needle. A solution containing a weakened a mount of the material being tested is injected into the skin. *Be aware that the injection itself causes a small bump to appear.* The area is checked for a reaction within 15 minutes. A test is considered, positive if the bump becomes swollen and red.

In both methods, a control test is done with a neutral solution which is usually the fluid used to dilute the materials being tested. The control test ideally does not cause a reaction because it contains no antigen material to cause an allergic reaction.

Almost every allergy sufferer who has ever sought professional help has encountered scratch or intradermal tests and been told that three to five years of treatment are necessary to relieve symptoms. The fact is that relief should occur in three to five months or the cause of the allergy has, not been correctly identified! The fact that most people expect to take allergy shots for three to five years shows how generally inaccurate scratch and intradermal tests really are. Let's see why.

First, even when skin tests prove accurate, they only show

that the skin is sensitive to that specific material. Just because the skin is sensitive does not necessarily mean the tissue which produces the symptoms (i.e., the area actually affected: the nose, lungs, stomach, or nervous system) will be sensitive to the same material!

Second, scratch and intracutaneous skin tests can create specific and nonspecific reactions. A specific reaction means the skin tissue has become swollen and red because it is allergic to the material being tested. A nonspecific reaction means the skin tissue has swollen and turned red for some reason other than an allergy. A nonspecific test falsely shows positive results. The point should be simple to grasp: both reactions look the same, but one has nothing to do with an allergy! Sound confusing? That is one reason skin tests are inaccurate. Mistakes can be made in deciding whether reactions are caused by allergies. More proof? Here it is. People can also show *positive test results* without having an allergy if the material being tested is too concentrated! And, remember, the material for tests usually comes in concentrated form. The kitchen of any good cook has vanilla extract and lemon in concentrate form. Right? Well, an allergist's laboratory or *kitchen* has extracts and concentrates of pollens, molds, house dust, insects, animal dander, and various foods. To avoid false reactions, the extract or testing material must be diluted. Mistakes can occur in the dilution process. Besides, the materials are not diluted to the same strengths all the time or even used consistently in the testing process. So, clearly, we have a double problem: materials must reach tissues in strong enough doses to cause allergic reactions and, at the same time, not be so strong that they cause spurious results.

With injection tests, the material is put inside different skin layers using a small hypodermic needle. It is difficult to control which layers of skin are to receive the injection. As you might

9

guess, shallow layers show greater reactions than deeper layers. The needle can also influence results. A ragged needlepoint that tears skin during an injection can easily cause a reaction (e.g., positive test) when no allergy exists at all! In short, skin tests are inaccurate for a lot of reasons.

On the other hand, provocative methods are much more accurate and form THE BASIS FOR THE BOOK YOU ARE READING. According to Webster's Dictionary, *provoke* comes from the Latin *pro* (forth) and *vocare* (to call) and means *to excite to some action or feeling; to anger or irritate; to stir up (action or feeling); to evoke.*

With provocative testing, the patient's allergic reaction or symptoms are literally *called forth.* Other methods depend on getting minor reactions, not actual symptoms. And *mistakes, as* I have discussed previously, can be made in evaluating the cause of an allergy based upon minor reactions. A test that produces actual symptoms leaves little doubt as to the cause. Many types of provocative tests can be used, but for now, we will consider one such test as an example. Others will be discussed in later chapters.

To test for materials that might cause an allergic reaction, that particular material is given to the patient in the office setting that might be inhaled by the patient in a real life situation. The powder of a particular material, such as from molds or pollens, is placed into one nostril while holding the other nostril closed. The powder enters the nose, throat, and airways to the lungs. By way of example, during the hay fever season, a person might inhale 1,000 pollen grains in 24 hours if the area had a pollen count of 1,200 or more. During the provocative test situation, a person would inhale 5,000 to 15,000 grains in a few seconds. A large amount of material comes in contact with sensitive nasal passages which makes this method extremely accurate. If the patient is allergic to the material being tested (placed on the end of a flat toothpick), a noticeable reaction occurs in less than five minutes with symptoms just like the patient has in real life. A nasal reaction usually involves sneezing, congestion, and a runny nose. A bronchial reaction involves coughing and wheezing. It's very simple: no sneeze, no wheeze, no allergy.

Once a reaction occurs, testing stops until the reaction is controlled. Symptoms usually can be relieved by spraying the nose with nose drops or inhaling a bronchial dilator which opens the airways to the lungs. After controlling the reaction, more tests can be made. Most patients can handle 20 to 30 tests in one sitting without difficulty.

Positive tests are repeated, but the order of materials tested is reversed. This eliminates the chance that materials negatively overlap, causing spurious results. A positive test confirmed by a second trial is highly accurate.

Many allergists feel that this type of testing should be done in a hospital, as they are concerned that the patient might go into shock from the sudden rush of *poison* material into the body. The danger is highly exaggerated. I have done more than 250,000 provocative nasal tests over a period of 20 years without encountering a single *dangerous reaction.* In support of my position and a further example, Dr. Marshall Mandell of Norwalk, Connecticut, has done thousands of such tests as well without any problems occurring. Further, I have induced many attacks of asthma ranging from minor to severe, and the symptoms produced by provocative testing are no worse than the symptoms many patients endure daily when they first enter an allergist's office for help. Such reactions are stopped by having the patient inhale a bronchial dilator from a nebulizer. At times, an injection of adrenalin is necessary to ease symptoms.

I compared the results of provocative nasal tests with those of scratch and intradermal tests. Proof of the provocative test's accuracy is presented in a later chapter. For now, we will assume that two positive tests (one reaction during regular testing and a second reaction during testing repeat) using my methods accurately indicate that the person is allergic to the tested material.

Let us look at some different test results comparing skin tests and provocative testing. The irritating agents were ragweed, ten different trees, two grasses, and 12 molds. Methods of test: scratch and injection. The patients were then retested using the provocative nasal tests. The following results are a matter of clinical record and can be produced at any time.

One hundred and sixty-seven people with nasal allergy were tested for ragweed. Forty positive reactions occurred with the scratch test and 81 using the injection method. No reaction occurred using either test in 46 patients.

The patients were then retested using provocative nasal tests. Of the 40 patients registering positive on the scratch tests, 35 had positive nasal tests and five had no reaction. A positive scratch test for ragweed pollen, then, is accurate 87.5 per cent of the time. That is, 12 to 13 patients out of 100 with positive scratch tests would receive unnecessary treatment for ragweed allergy if treatment was based only on scratch tests. While this is not a bad percentage, the alarming fact remains: far too few patients register positive scratch tests when they are indeed allergic!

However, of the 81 who had positive injection tests for ragweed, only 48 had positive nasal tests. The injection tests for ragweed, then, are accurate only 59.2 per cent of the time! That is, 41 out of 100 patients would receive useless treatment, if such treatment was based solely on an injection test.

The reliability of skin tests varies depending on the method used. The scratch test is accurate, or relatively so, for ragweed, but detecting allergies to trees is a different story. Ten patients who had 24 positive tests to trees (i.e., some patients are allergic to more than one kind of tree), only 12 had positive sniff tests. When it comes to trees, the scratch test is only accurate half the time! Injection tests for tree allergies are almost useless. Of 400 positive injection tests, nasal testing only confirmed 97 reactions. Injection tests for tree allergies are accurate, then, less than one-fourth of the time! That means 75 out of 100 patients with positive injection tests for tree pollens receive unnecessary treatment (assumes an accuracy rate of less than 25 per cent). The general rule of thumb in medicine is that any treatment should attain a 75 per cent accuracy, or it is not considered an effective cure. Referring to the 400 positive injection tests, that accuracy rate runs right around 25 per cent, a rather poor showing. Another way to look at it: those 75 patients would be treated for tree allergies for three to five years when they are really allergic to something else.

The intracutaneous tests for molds showed equal dismal findings. These tests in a large number of patients were correct only 26 per cent of the time. Thus, 74 out of 100 patients would get needless treatment for molds.

Scratch tests are quite efficient of what they show, but far too few patients show enough of a positive reaction to allow successful treatment. As a result, many allergists have discontinued scratch tests and rely only on injection tests. Injection tests are highly inaccurate, as they give false *positives* leading to needless treatment.

There have been some reports that provocative nasal tests and intracutaneous tests had a good clinical accuracy. These reports are based upon the use of nasal aerosol sprays. One report many years ago was based upon the production of symptoms such as sneezing, congestion, and drainage. thoroughly checked out this type of testing and found it to be very nonspecific. One day symptoms would occur and, when checked the next day, the symptoms were absent or, in a sense, the patients exhibited different types of symptoms. Clearly, this is of no value.

Again, in more recent years, provocative nasal testing with aerosol sprays, either with a nebulizer or drops of allergy extracts, has been used, with localized reactions usually checked up to one hour periods. Claims have been made that visible reactions in the nasal mucous membranes checked out well with the skin tests. The fact is that any spray or drops on the nasal lining of the nose will cause some nonspecific reactions. The extracts used are of an allergic or nonallergenic nature. To be accurate, symptoms must be produced similar to those which occur in the allergic patient! The next chapter clarifies this point.

# 3

# *PROVOCATIVE SKIN TESTS FOR DIAGNOSIS OF INHALANT ALLERGENS*

Patients whose treatment is based upon provocative nasal tests respond better than patients whose treatment is based upon traditional skin tests. However, many variables influence clinical results and, as such, this experience alone does not prove the superiority of the sniff tests described in the last chapter. To verify the accuracy of nasal tests, I did provocative skin tests and compared those results with the results of sniff tests and patient symptoms.

Provocative skin tests have the same objectives as provocative nasal tests: to create the symptoms the patient has in real life and to pinpoint the cause of the allergy. A provocative skin test differs from the traditional skin tests described in the previous chapter. With provocative skin tests for inhalants (things people breathe that cause allergies), a weak solution of an allergy-causing material or allergen is injected into the deep layers of the skin. A weak solution is used at first to avoid a severe reaction, followed by progressively more concentrated solutions. If a patient is allergic to the material, he will react with one or more of his usual symptoms within 20 minutes. Those symptoms may be asthma, sneezing, coughing, hives, nasal congestion, and discharge. This method is highly accurate and produces a reaction if an allergy is present.

If the weak solution does not produce a reaction, a second injection approximately ten times stronger than the first is made. If this test does not create a reaction, a third injection is made ten times stronger than the second. If negative, a fourth injection of the strongest or stock extract is made. If the last injection does not produce symptoms in 40 minutes, the patient is not allergic to the material tested.

Using a variety of allergy-causing agents, provocative skin tests were conducted on 180 patients who had responded with 351 positive reactions to nasal or sniff tests of differing materials. People who had 147 positive sniff tests for molds had 132 positive reactions to provocative injection tests, meaning that treatment for molds based upon provocative nasal tests is 90 per cent accurate. That means only 10 per cent of the people having positive sniff tests would have received unnecessary treatment. Whereas, with skin tests, 74 per cent would have received needless treatment.

Provocative injection tests for dust produced 154 reactions in the 162 people who had positive nasal tests. That means sniff tests for dust are accurate 95 per cent of the time! That is, only 5 patients out of 100 would have received unnecessary treatment based upon nasal tests.

Of 12 patients that nasal tests showed to be sensitive to grass, provocative injection-test reactions confirmed 11 cases. The nasal tests for grasses is therefore 92 per cent accurate. Nasal tests proved 100 per cent accurate in detecting ragweed allergies.

HOWEVER, IDENTIFYING A SINGLE CAUSE OF AN ALLERGIC REACTION DOES NOT MEAN A CURE IS AT HAND. Successful treatment for the allergic patient depends upon uncovering ALL irritating substances. If the patient is allergic to ten substances and eight of those are diagnosed in testing and treated, the patient will not necessarily be 80 per cent better! The patient surely may be only slightly improved because the two substances missed in testing may be the major causes of the patient's true illness. April Simmons of Galveston, Texas, a ten-year-old girl who was receiving treatment elsewhere based upon traditional scratch and injection tests, is a good example of this very crucial point. April had been receiving therapy for over a year without relief. She still had the classic symptoms such as congestion, a runny nose, and occasional sneezing. April was being treated for allergies to dust, molds, and pollens. April's mother was not overly concerned about the symptoms because she had been told, by the allergist April was seeing at the time, that three years of treatment could be expected as necessary for her daughter's relief. One of my patients (a friend of April's mother), suggested that the family come and see me, that I considered any treatment a failure if no relief occurred within three to five months. That was the situation under which April and her mother first came to visit and an examination was conducted.

April did not react to any materials using provocative nasal tests, indicating she was not allergic to materials she breathed and despite the positive reactions to the traditional skin tests held at the office of her former allergist. I recommended admitting April to St. Mary Hospital and stopped all food for three days, a therapeutic fasting which is the subject of a later chapter. April completely recovered and showed no symptoms after three days of fasting. She then ate a single, different food at three-hour intervals during the day, challenge feeding which also is discussed in a later chapter.

April reacted positively to ten different foods tested. She was discharged from the hospital with a diet omitting the ten irritating foods and has remained well to this day. Point: foods were the sole cause of April's allergies and not the inhalants for which she had previously been treated.

# 4

# *PROVOCATIVE OPHTHALMIC TESTING*

The key to successful allergy treatment is properly identifying the cause of the allergy. The logic to provocative testing is simple: *produce the allergic reaction (eg., wheezing in the chest) and you've identified the cause of the allergy. No* reaction means you keep looking.

Other provocative tests can be performed such as ophthalmic or eye tests and food tests. The provocative test of choice depends upon the allergy and material being tested. Provocative eye tests have been used for years by a very few allergists, especially to detect pollen sensitivity. The test is highly accurate, and it is a good way to confirm mixed results of nasal tests. Yet, most allergists do not include it in their testing repertory, preferring instead less accurate skin tests. The eye's mucous membrane is similar to that of the respiratory tract. When the nasal and bronchial membranes are sensitive to allergens, the conjunctiva or eye membrane is usually sensitive as well. When a true positive provocative nasal test occurs, the eye also reacts positively to the same substance.

However, a positive eye test does not necessarily mean a positive nasal test!

Sheila Barnes, a 16-year-old student-athlete from Houston, Texas, had conjunctivitis, an inflammation of the eye membrane, but she had no nasal symptoms during the spring months. Confusing? It was. Nasal pollens proved negative as was expected, but Sheila's eye reacted markedly to Italian and perennial rye grass pollen. Specific therapy for these pollens produced excellent results. She was allergic all right, but her nasal tissues were not sensitive to the pollens.

A positive eye test proves the eye is sensitive. It does not prove the allergen responsible for the positive test is the specific cause of all bronchial or nasal symptoms when an individual is allergic to more than one substance. A patient may be sensitive to four substances or allergens, and all may cause symptoms. One may cause only bronchial symptoms, another nasal and bronchial symptoms, a third only nasal symptoms, and the fourth eye and nasal symptoms. When only a few allergens are involved, specificity is necessary to reach a successful diagnosis. To successfully treat allergy and eliminate all symptoms, all the causes of the allergy must be properly identified. That is why provocative testing is so successful and why traditional methods fall way short.

The success of nasal or sniff tests were discussed previously. Should nasal tests prove truly inconclusive, an eye test should be done. If the eye test is negative, almost without exception that means the nasal test is negative or, at the very least, nonspecific.

If you have been following along carefully, then you should be at the point of asking the very telling question: IF EYE TESTS ARE SO ACCURATE, WHY NOT RELY ON THEM ALL THE TIME? The answer to that intrigue is, very simply, that the eye is extremely sensitive. The eye test involves taking a small amount of the powdered allergen being tested and placing it on the inner surface of the lower eye lid. If a reaction does not occur within five minutes, the test is negative. Negative tests do not cause discomfort, and a number of tests can be performed at one sitting. However, positive tests can be irritating. At the first sign of a reaction (redness, itching, and tearing of the eye), the allergen is removed with a cotton swab and the eye flushed with a few drops of Epinephrine to stop the reaction. Too long a delay can cause moderate discomfort. The potential for discomfort is the problem with eye tests.

Although extremely accurate and very specific, eye tests can be very irritating, which makes repeated use difficult if even a few positive reactions occur. On the other hand, positive nasal tests are less irritating, so additional nasal tests can readily be conducted even if many tests are positive.

Since the patient's comfort and well-being are of utmost importance, nasal tests are the method of choice in most cases involving the testing of powdered allergens. However, eye tests are valuable for verifying questionable nasal test results. The eye tests also should be used to test allergens not available in powdered form because the heavy particles are not readily inhaled. House dust mites, for example, are microscopic insects, a source of allergy for many people. If not tested in powdered form, the particles are too heavy to enter the bronchial tubes so that reactions don't occur with nasal tests.

When insect allergens are in powdered form, positive nasal tests should be verified with eye tests. Powdered insects (cockroaches, spiders, crickets, and red ants) are less specific in nasal tests than molds and pollens. The reliability of eye and nasal tests done as a unit have been confirmed with provocative skin tests, which are as close to 100 per cent accurate as can be imagined.

# 5

# *PROVOCATIVE TESTING FOR DIAGNOSIS OF FOOD ALLERGY*

Provocative testing for food allergies is possible. I used different methods of such testing for some time, and these efforts helped develop the method I now use.

In 1963, 1 used a method developed by Rinkel which called for injecting food extracts into the superficial layers of the skin to produce symptoms in patients allergic to specific foods. This method was more accurate in diagnosing food allergy than traditional skin tests, but the test itself caused local discomfort, thus making it impractical for testing children. I substituted provocative skin tests in which the allergen is injected under the skin. This method worked as well and caused less local discomfort. The goal, though, was to find the most accurate test possible while at the same time causing the least amount of discomfort. Switching to sublingual tests in which drops of food extract were placed under the patient's tongue proved as effective as the skin tests and caused no local discomfort.

With each of the three methods just described, a positive test produced symptoms similar to that which patients had experienced in real life, such as nasal congestion, coughing, post nasal drip, asthma, headaches, fatigue, gastrointestinal discomfort and hives. The problem, though, was that the patients needed to be completely free of symptoms before the tests had any real accuracy. At that point, then, positive tests were highly diagnostic, but negative tests still had to be confirmed by challenge feeding the particular food to the patient. The big discovery was that only 35 to 49 per cent accurate, way below the 75 per cent level needed to be of any real value.

Although I no longer use these methods in my practice to diagnose food allergy, the knowledge gained in testing and documenting their accuracy has pointed the way in the technique of therapeutic fasting and challenge feeding which is highly accurate, and which I now use exclusively to diagnose food allergies. This method was pioneered by Dr. Theron Randolph. Since foods are the culprits for many allergies and related physical discomfort symptoms, more so than many traditional allergists would like to imagine, an entire separate chapter in this book is devoted to that specific topic.

# 6

# THE PATIENT'S HISTORY AS RELATED TO THE DIAGNOSIS OF ALLERGY

Doctors who use traditional testing methods in attempting to pinpoint sources of allergy have necessarily had to compensate for the inaccuracy and inefficiency of those methods. The most common tool in use is the *patient history,* and no discussion of allergy diagnosis is complete without considering the value of this procedure.

Any competent physician takes a patient history, as otherwise he might prescribe a treatment of medication that, for example, conflicts with a medication the patient is already taking, fails to consider childhood diseases, or does not take into account a family's tendency toward heart disease or diabetes. A proper history forms the foundation upon which the doctor builds his case diagnosis and subsequent treatment plan.

However, some allergists attach so much importance to *the patient history* that it seems to take on a life of its own. Such reliance on histories occurs because of the poor diagnostic results obtained with traditional skin tests, which makes *history taking* sort of a last-chance stop. These allergists spend lengthy sessions with patients going over their histories and trying to determine the cause of the allergic symptoms. These allergists rely on factors of inheritance, food intolerances, emotional stresses, and other possible influences. Some allergists even treat patients based upon histories alone! For example, after an initial lengthy history taking, additional sessions may be necessary in the allergist's relentless search for a reasonable diagnosis, as the allergist gropes over his notes and wonders if the patient left out some important detail concerning the patient's grandmother or father's side of the family. A recurring allergy that gets worse at given times of the year casts suspicion on pollens as the allergen. It may also provide information on the relationship of symptoms to certain seasonal foods, activities, and living habits.

The ongoing history may suggest a relationship between symptoms and the work place, marriage, divorce, death of a mate, or any exciting or depressing event which may mean physical symptoms are occurring as a reaction to emotional distress. Incidence of respiratory infections may mean a connection with bacterial allergy, and attacks at night may indicate some article of bedding or item in the bedroom is the cause. The details of history taking varies with different allergists, but the goal is the same: A RELENTLESS AND, TOO OFTEN, HOPELESS SEARCH FOR A DIAGNOSTIC MIRACLE.

Fact: no amount of history taking can give a complete or even near complete answer to any case of perennial or recurring allergy whether of the respiratory tract, central nervous system, gastrointestin al tract, skin, or any combination of the four areas.

True, a history of seasonal allergy lasting a month or two casts suspicion on pollens, but it cannot exact the specific pollen or pollens causing the problem from the season's many active pollens.

Make no mistake about it: a history is a necessary procedure. A long history, though, adds little useful knowledge in diagnosing allergy *while adding greatly to the allergist's fee.*

Foods are an important element in perennial allergy involving 75 per cent of perennial allergic patients. However, few patients believe or suspect they have a food allergy! The patients who do suspect foods may identify one or two foods that cause trouble but rarely can identify all the foods that occupy a place in the allergic picture. Compare the results of provocative types of testing with the findings of a detailed patient history. IT IS EASY TO SEE HOW THE DETAILED HISTORY APPROACH RESULTS IN PATIENT FRUSTRATION AND FALSE HOPE.

Moreover, histories are important but only as the foundation for provocative testing. The allergist should make certain the patient does not overlook a chronic history of post nasal drip, sniffing, clearing of the throat after eating, morning hacking and hawking to clear the throat, headaches, gastrointestinal symptoms and other recurring problems. Many cigarette smokers brush off upper respiratory problems as resulting from tobacco. Patients with headaches and stomach problems brush off these irritations with self-made diagnoses of *nerves or tension.*

A rough estimate of symptoms' duration in months or years is important. If there is nasal involvement, it is important to know if the patient is using nose drops and hypertension drugs. A significant number of chronic nasal congestion cases have been cleared up by stopping the use of nose drops and hypertension drugs. My son, for example, used a nose spray for relief of cold symptoms. Over time, he developed the habit of using the drops every night to help him breathe more easily while sleeping. The spray did open his nasal passages, but it also had a rebound effect. As the spray wore off, the nasal passages became even more blocked. The spray was causing the congestion, not an allergy! Once he broke away from the spray bottle dependency, the congestion disappeared!

A perfect example of unwanted side effects for improperly prescribed drugs comes form they case of Rob Hill, a middle-aged, Westinghouse quality control engineer from Chicago, Illinois, who came into my office one day while on a business trip to the Houston, Texas area. He had been suffering from chronic nasal congestion for about three years. It happened that a side effect of Bob's blood pressure medication was nasal congestion. Allergy tests were not done at this time, but the blood pressure medication was stopped. Bob was told to report back to my office in ten days. By that time he was completely well! A new hypertension drug was started with perfect results and no side effects. In addition, an ancillary point to be made here deals with headaches and related symptoms. The presence of headaches and related symptoms may lead to a diagnosis of histamine, migraine, tension or allergic headache, but every so-called *tension headache* should be considered allergic until diagnosed otherwise.

Moreover, the presence of gastrointestinal symptoms and chronic edema or swelling, especially of the hands and feet in the morning, may well point to an allergy. A history of gallstones and peptic ulcers, supported by x-rays continue to cause problems in spite of medical and surgical treatment, is strong evidence of an allergy. This is especially significant in recurring ulcers.

Asking questions about general health, anemia and thyroid deficiency are important matters in any patient history survey, as well as questions dealing with the home heating system and type of bedding (e.g., foam rubber or feather pillows). And, certainly, questions dealing with live-in home pets should be considered routine. An aggravation of symptoms, such as when the person enters a particular type of store such as a fabric shop or auto tire store, is important information. A history of bedding material and especially pillow-material composition is very important. If the patient has nasal congestion and/or wheezing during the night and in the morning but gets moderate or even complete relief after leaving the bedroom, these are absolute indicators of an allergy to the dacron or feather pillow. Substituting a cotton pillow or two works wonders. After only a single night, relief is obtained if the pillow is a factor. In my office, I keep six new cotton pillows at all times. If a patient has night and early morning symptoms, I loan the patient a couple of pillows for use that night. If relief occurs, the patient keeps the pillows and is on the road to recovery. If relief is not immediate, the patient returns the pillows, and we continue to search for a solution. This routine has cleared many patients of some or all of their allergy symptoms. This procedure is simple, thoughtful, and requires only a little imagination. If this particular case history fits you, give it a chance. A miracle just might occur.

In my office, this initial patient history investigation takes about 20 minutes or so. Provocative testing then starts in a room that seats 12 patients. As testing proceeds and as the patient converses with other patients, significant bits of history emerge that the patient perhaps forgot and might never recall, regardless of how long the duration of the patient history inventory might have taken. For example, Mary Stuart, of Austin, Texas, a car rental clerk at the Municipal Airport, claimed no contact with dogs or cats. She reacted with violent sneezing after provocative nasal tests executed with cat hair. She then recalled sneezing a lot when playing Rook (a card game similar to Bridge) at a friend's house. The friend's cat always prowled under the card table, and Mary often would stroke the cat. The information was dormant in her mind, but positive tests brought instant recall.

# 7

# *RELATIONSHIP OF IMMUNIZATION AND HYPOSENSITIZATION IN CLINICAL ALLERGY*

The provocative testing procedure is clearly the most reliable method available for identifying the cause of allergy. However, now that we know the cause of an allergy, how do we treat the allergy and how successful is that treatment likely to be? In short, what's all this talk about allergy shots, and do they work?

Fact: not all allergies need to be treated with shots. The best way to control allergies is simply to avoid the substance or allergen causing the allergic reaction. Easy enough if the patient is allergic to pineapple. But it is not so easy if the patient is allergic to something in the air, and as we all know oxygen is necessary to sustain life on earth as we know it. The patient simply can't avoid breathing to solve the problem and will need injections to help build up a tolerance to the offending substance. Yes, shots do work, but only if the specific cause has been properly identified. Then, and only then, will the patient be free of symptoms in three to five months. However, most allergists don't get such positive results. Why? BECAUSE INADEQUACY OF THEIR TESTING METHODS ULTIMATELY YIELD POOR TREATMENT THERAPY! A specific discussion regarding food allergy treatment is contained in the chapter on food allergies. But, remember, all allergies have one thing in common: they involve sensitive tissue reacting to the presence of an irritating substance or allergic stimulus which produces symptoms. *Sensitive* as used in this context does not mean delicate to handle. It means susceptible to reaction. For example, Mr. Jones handles poison ivy and is not affected by it, while Mr. Smith handles the same plant and breaks out in a severe rash. Mr. Smith is simply sensitive to poison ivy while Mr. Jones is not.

In allergy patients, these sensitized or shock tissues react because of the presence of sensitizing antibodies. The nasal passages as shock tissue may produce symptoms of sneezing, discharge, or blockage. The lungs as shock tissue may respond with coughing and wheezing. The brain may react with headaches, depression, sluggishness, or hyperactivity. Any part of the body may react to an allergen if that part is sensitized.

The ultimate goal of clinical allergy treatment is the complete desensitization of the various shock tissues. If this can be accomplished, the sensitized shock tissue loses its sensitivity and becomes incapable of producing allergic symptoms, and the patient, then, is effectively cured.

The path toward the cure involves allergy shots, injections of antigens of the offending substances. The antigens cause the patient's body to react by producing antibodies to fight the invading substances. The more antibodies the patient produces, the greater is the tolerance against the offending substance, and immunity takes place.

The importance of identifying the specific cause of an allergic reaction should be obvious. Provocative testing methods do so with great accuracy, and this explains my personal success in treating allergy patients for the past 20 years. Traditional testing methods and patient histories are, for obvious reasons, unreliable in diagnosing allergies, and so are the treatments prescribed based upon those methods. This leads us to one of the most misunderstood concepts in allergy today. IMMUNIZATION IS NOT THE SAME AS DESENSITIZATION!

When an injection of an antigen is given, the body produces blocking antibodies almost immediately, although it takes three or four days to get measurable amounts in the blood. This antibody production leads to immunization just as a shot of tetanus vaccine yields protection or immunity against that disease. When a sufficiently high concentration level of blocking antibodies is reached, they will neutralize the specific allergen or substance introduced into the system much like a vaccine enables the body to destroy invading germs.

Allergy shots primarily produce immunization, and a high degree of immunization is not necessarily followed by an equal degree of desensitization. Even though the patient has not been desensitized, he can expect his symptoms to disappear with immunization. The success of the immunization can be checked with a provocative test. If the patient reacted to a diluted substance such as mold extract before treatment and does not react to the same test after receiving injections, a good immunity has been achieved. However, if treatment is not continued, this immunity or protection will be lost within a few months or more and symptoms will recur when the patient is exposed to the offending substance. This is an example of the patient being immune *not desensitized*.

The treatment does, in some or even most cases, produce desensitization in time. That means the shock tissue is no longer sensitive to this particular allergen. Provocative nasal tests will confirm that the patient is no longer sensitive to concentrated does of the allergen. The cure may last for months or years. No one really knows why one individual is only immunized while another is desensitized.

But this is not the whole story, either. Some years ago, I treated Tanya Bangston, a ten-year-old girl who lived in the San Antonio area. Tanya had moderately severe recurring asthma and nasal allergy during the period of time where I still did not seriously apply provocative testing in my allergy practice. Tanya had a positive scratch test to house dust. All other tests were negative. A year on dust therapy failed to eliminate symptoms. Her mother took her elsewhere, and that allergist, as well, treated her with house dust therapy for another year, and without benefit. Tanya returned to me about the time I introduced provocative nasal testing as a substitute for skin testing. Using provocative testing on two different days, she had a marked bronchial and nasal reaction to only one antigen, a mold called *stemphyllium botrytis*. Therapy with this one mold produced a clinical cure! After two years of therapy, Tanya's mother wanted to stop treatment. A provocative nasal test was repeated with the powdered mold, and the patient again had a marked reaction. Tanya had been clinically cured due to excellent immunization, but she had not been clinically desensitized. Tanya continued therapy for another year. The provocative nasal test was repeated and no reaction occurred. Tanya, now, had been immunized as well as desensitized. Tanya was discharged, and she remained well for two years. At that time, symptoms returned. A provocative nasal test for the mold was negative! Obviously, she had developed new sensitivities. A complete allergic survey was done. Tanya had developed allergies to eight foods! Symptoms disappeared once these foods were removed from her diet.

Once a patient has been successfully immunized, rather than desensitized, that person will be symptom-free while living in a normal environment. But if a patient is allergic, say, to house dust

33

mites and goes into an attic where old mattresses are stored, symptoms will probably occur and be quite severe because of the excessive amount of house dust mite antigen that is inhaled. This acute circumstance amounts to a real provocative nasal test! Once the patient leaves the attic, the symptoms will not last because the amount of antigen reaching the bloodstream will be neutralized by the blocking antibodies. If there was no immunity, such an exposure might result in an asthma attack lasting for several days rather than a few hours.

The amount of most antigens invading the respiratory tract under normal living conditions will not cause an immediate reaction. But if exposure to the antigen continues, the bloodstream absorbs the inhaled antigen. Eventually, enough antigen has accumulated to overpower the immune antibodies and produce a severe allergic reaction. Remove the patient from the area with the offending antigen, and the amount of antigen in the patient's system will be exhausted in two or three days and symptoms will cease.

Moreover, a patient may have built up enough immunity to dog dander to have a small pet without the person experiencing allergic reactions. However, going over to Aunt Sally's house to baby-sit her three dogs for the weekend may cause an allergic reaction. The patient has overstepped his immunity by about two dogs' worth! The good news, though, is when the patient goes back to a one-dog routine at home the symptoms disappear.

Important point: *ragweed* is a notable exception to all this immunization and desensitization talk. *Ragweed* is such a toxic antigen that, in areas with high concentrations of *ragweed,* no level of immunity prevents all symptoms. A patient must achieve desensitization before any real relief is experienced from the *ragweed pollen.* I personally know of colleagues who say they have achieved excellent relief of *ragweed* allergy symptoms in most patients subjected to shots. I asked one such allergist what the *ragweed pollen* count was in his area, New York City. He said as high as 100. I don't doubt he has gotten such results in his neighborhood. However, my practice is located in southeastern Texas where *ragweed pollen* counts are typically 1,200 during the high season! Any allergist could get positive results from *ragweed pollen* therapy for pollen counts of 100! Few allergists can get positive results from pollen counts of 1,200 unless desensitization has been accomplished.

Generally, injection therapy is successful for pollens, molds, house dust mites, and foods. Each antigen, though, has its own peculiar  characteristics and is more effective in some cases than in others. The first program of injection therapy was introduced more than 60 years ago by an allergist named Cooke, who gave weekly injections. His method consisted of starting with a weak antigen solution, gradually increasing the strength of the extract according to the patient's tolerance. The method pioneered by Cooke remains the allergy treatment of choice.

The purpose of this type of therapy is to increase the patient's immunity by stimulating the immune mechanism, thus producing blocking antibodies. The stronger the dose of antigenic extract the patient can tolerate, the greater the immunity. The treatment's success depends upon the patient's sensitivity, tolerance level, and the toxicity of the allergen.

# 8

# *RESULTS OF THERAPY*
# *TRUE OR FALSE*

Traditional allergists employing traditional methods claim that 60 to 70 per cent of their patients are helped by desensitizing injections. Crucial point: there is little doubt that such a percentage of patients *will say* they have achieved satisfactory results, meaning that they are *better* than before therapy! But this condition can be misleading. In many cases, as a result of chance or adaptation (e.g., patient adjusting to his surroundings), the allergy sufferer is responsible for the improvement, not the specific therapy. As noted in a previous chapter, treatment based upon patient histories and skin tests has a diagnostic efficiency of 25 to 40 per cent, meaning that 60 to 75 patients out of 100 receive worthless treatment. Proof: the role of chance or adaptation is easily proved by studies in which patients were given no specific therapy at all!

Perhaps it is time to cite a number of case studies to more fully support the above conclusions. Buffum and Asettipone studied 518 asthma patients for ten years to examine the effects of the illness. After that period, the researchers concluded that 42 per cent of the patients had no symptoms; 52.4 per cent had slight or occasional symptoms; and 5.6 per cent had enough asthmatic symptom identification to be considered handicapped. Johnstone studied 91 asthmatic children for four years. During that time, 18 per cent became free of asthma and 22.2 per cent lost accompanying asthmatic symptoms by the time they turned 16 years old. In a five-year study of 95 children, Montgomery and Smith showed that 75 per cent had much less trouble while 30 per cent had no asthma attacks at all during the last year of the examination time period. Between 60 and 70 per cent of any patient group given weekly injections of sterile water for a year, accompanied by treatment of symptoms and an encouraging pat on the back, will say they are better! In many studies, placebo injections account for an improvement in 30 per cent of the patients. Now, throw in some sort of treatment for symptoms and one easily increases the *improvement* rate to as much as 70 per cent. But frequently the injection therapy based upon the *Holy Trinity* of dust, molds, and pollens gets the credit. The only result that means anything should be that the patient is well or near well within three to five months of treatment by correctly identifying the cause of the allergens and eliminating the problem, NOT MERELY PRESCRIBING JUST ABOUT ANYTHING TO THE PATIENT FROM PLACEBOS TO M&M'S TO TREAT THE SYMPTOMS.

Without question, traditional allergists do achieve some successes with the *Holy Trinity* approach, generally falling into the category of seasonal allergies. These allergists arrive at the proper therapy using a shotgun approach. A positive intracutaneous test for pollens is only 30 per cent accurate. The traditional allergist then begins treatment for the broad spectrum of pollens. This means that no pollens affecting the patient will be omitted from treatment, but, as well, many pollens that don't cause symptoms will be included. When unnecessary antigens are included in the treatment mixture, the patient is not likely to receive doses of the important proper antigens in levels high enough to achieve maximum immunity.

Using provocative testing methods, the specific allergen can be readily identified and the appropriate antigen prescribed. While traditional allergists give injections week after week, another more appropriate regime is highly satisfactory. In order to obtain faster immunity, two injections weekly can be administered for the first two or three weeks while increasing the strength of the antigen extract. Then, weekly injections can be given until the concentrated dilution is properly reached. If this dose is tolerated without symptoms or undue local reactions, the maintenance dose is reached at 0.1 **cc** of the concentrated extract. After two months of weekly injections of this dose, the time interval is reduced to one injection every two weeks for two or three months. Then, monthly injections are given, sufficient to maintain immunity and are more convenient and cost effective for the patient.

# 9

# *POLLENS IN ALLERGY*

The body is a relatively closed system, and we are fairly well protected against invasion from harmful substances in the outside world, until, of course, we breathe or put something in our mouths. Since we have little choice about breathing or eating to stay alive, it should be no surprise that our nose and mouth are the principal ways in which harmful allergic substances enter the body.

Inhalants and their effects have been previously discussed. Now, we will take a closer look at those things that can cause allergies when people breathe. Food allergies will be discussed in a later chapter.

Dust, molds, and pollens are the most common causes of inhalant-related allergies. Inhalant allergies can manifest themselves in other ways, but they typically enter the body through and impact the respiratory system. For example, nasal allergy is a common ailment affecting millions of people throughout the world. Symptoms are nasal congestion, postnasal drip, headaches, pain over the nasal and sinus areas, and, in general, feeling of pressure in affected areas. When sneezing is the predominant symptom, the condition is commonly called hay fever which is due to an air-borne pollen. Pretty flowers, quite simply, are not the culprits many people might think. Those flashy flowers are pollinated by insects. The pollen is too heavy to float for more than a short distance before falling to the ground. Plants such as roses will cause sneezing only when a sensitive person passes nearby or deliberately sniffs them. Pollens from grasses, weeds, and trees are responsible for most nasal allergy, and all too often traditional allergists incorrectly blame them for causing nasal symptoms and even asthma.

The more pollens present in the air, the more severe the hay fever symptoms. In addition to sneezing, those all too familiar symptoms immortalized in television commercials can involve tearing of the eyes, nasal congestion, nasal and eye itching and headaches. Symptoms are worse in the early morning hours when trees, weeds, and grasses tend to release their pollens.

While the traditional allergist talks about pollen asthma, it rarely occurs. Occasionally, symptoms of severe hay fever are followed by a mild asthma. As a result of hundreds of provocative nasal tests with ragweed pollen conducted in my office over the years, a mild wheezing occurred in only two patients, persons who indeed did have mild asthma along with severe hay fever during the ragweed season. To impact the lungs and produce an asthma reaction, the allergen must reach the sensitive lung tissue. Ragweed pollen measures 15 microns (a single micron is 1/25,000 of an inch) and readily enters the bronchioles or airways of the lung which have 25 micron openings. Other tree and grass pollens are 25 microns or larger and are, therefore, too large to enter the bronchioles. They also do not produce lung symptoms with provocative nasal testing. Provocative skin tests conducted in my office on more than 100 hay fever patients who were sensitive to grass and tree pollens produced only nasal symptoms WITHOUT ASTHMA.

Using only traditional testing methods, diagnosing patients with active hay fever symptoms can result in false positive indicators. That is, patients with active hay fever may find their symptoms getting worse when they are exposed to animal dander, dust, and other common allergens. This does not mean the patient is allergic to these materials. It does mean that irritated tissues react to any foreign substance that makes its way into bodily systems! To determine actual allergic indices to these and any other possible allergens, tests must be done when the hay fever IS NOT ACTIVE. Quite clearly, tests may confirm that the patient is not allergic to preconceived suspected materials.

Studies conducted in my office over the years indicate that 30 per cent of patients with perennial respiratory allergy (year-round symptoms) are allergic to pollens. Ragweed is the primary culprit. So, remove this one pollen and the incidence of pollen allergy in perennial cases drops to 15 per cent. The pollens, of course, are only responsible for the nasal symptoms that occur during the pollen season. The good news and haven for ragweed sufferers is west of the Rocky Mountains where the plant doesn't grow. Otherwise, ragweed sufferers can expect to sneeze from this critter at least part of the year.

While on the subject, sneezing can actually be an important indicator in allergy diagnosis. For example, pollens are usually not responsible for nasal allergy symptoms IF THOSE SYMPTOMS DO NOT INCLUDE SNEEZING (especially if the symptoms occur throughout the year). When the nasal allergy symptoms are congestion, post nasal drip, and headache and sinus pressure with no sneezing, pollens can practically be ruled out as the cause. In these cases, the cause generally is due to molds, animal dander, food allergies, or a combination of these factors. When nasal symptoms with sneezing occur throughout the year, studies conducted in my office have shown that house dust mites, foods, molds or animal dander, with or without pollens, were the cause in a vast majority of cases.

However, in far too many cases, traditional allergists treat for pollen allergy without justification. Traditional skin test results are misleading and allergists who rely exclusively on them will necessarily assume that 60 to 80 per cent of their perennial nasal allergy patients are sensitive to pollens. As discussed earlier, tests indicate that pollens figure dominantly in only 30 per cent of the cases surveyed. This significant discrepancy in actual percentages cited above results from inherent testing inadequacy used by traditional allergists, thus not producing a reliability factor inherent in provocative testing. And, as stated previously, traditional intracutaneous skin tests are only 30 per cent accurate. In comparison, provocative nasal tests are 90 per cent accurate; this statement has been confirmed by Dr. Marshall Mandell of Norwalk, Connecticut, in his work on provocative nasal testing. Simply put, this means that, when traditional skin tests are used, 70 out of 100 patients receive needless treatment for pollens! However, when provocative tests are used, 90 per cent of patients treated receive effective cure.

# 10

## *MOLDS IN ALLERGY*

Molds are airborne materials that cause allergic reactions when inhaled by susceptible people. Molds are a misunderstood and critical cause of allergy, and, while there are many different varieties, only a few are actually responsible for allergic symptoms.

Molds grow best under warm, humid conditions. That is why they are prevalent in humid climates, especially in the warm Gulf region of the southeastern United States. In cold areas, molds are seasonal, occur in late spring, summer, and early fall. In warmer regions, incidence occurs throughout the year but tends to be most active in the spring and fall when humidity is higher.

Molds have exotic sounding names such as *Hormodendrum, Curvularia, and Phoma,* but from the patient's point of view what they are called is less important than the culprit's effects. Studies by Sorenson, Bulmer, and Criep show that molds occur throughout the United States and Puerto Rico with some variations but almost equal frequency. The most common molds fall into 14 distinct varieties. Provocative nasal testing shows that the most common molds are not necessarily ones causing the most problems for allergy sufferers. Several uncommon molds occurring in relatively small numbers provoked positive test results far more frequently than more common mold varieties. What is of real consequence here is how allergic the patient is to a given mold or molds, not the *commonness* of the mold itself. Small numbers of a particular mold can cause severe problems for someone who is extremely sensitive to it, and, conversely, large amounts of that same mold will cause no trouble at all unless the patient proves correspondingly sensitive.

It is true that a good patient history may suggest tracing the allergy source to molds. However, the patient history cannot isolate the mold or molds causing the trouble and should not be relied upon to make a diagnosis of mold allergy! Mold counts and plate exposures are frequently done in patient homes to determine which molds are present in the given environment. This method, though, is expensive and does not prove that the patient is sensitive to the molds found! Provocative nasal tests can accurately determine exactly which molds cause the specific allergic reactions being observed in the patient. Extensive mold testing using the 23 most common molds of the local area was done in my office in southeast Texas. After carefully studying the test results, it was determined that every patient with mold allergy was allergic to one or more molds in the *Dematiaceae* group (a group of six molds). Further, if a patient did not have a reaction to tests in this group, then tests for the other 17 common molds never caused a reaction! The significance of this finding should be quite clear. If no positive reaction occurred using the *Dematiaceae* group, then molds were not the cause of the allergic reaction! This may sound simple, but, to the traditional allergist, climbing this mountain can be almost an insurmountable task. Clearly, the method is accurate and saves wear and tear on the patient. Similarly, if a positive reaction is found to one of the group molds, then the patient is treated for all six. Why?

Experience has shown that treating for only one or a few of the six molds frequently results in the recurrence of symptoms as the patient develops sensitivity to other molds in the group.

Injection therapy can only go so far, and, in spite of an accurate diagnosis in mold allergy, results may be found somewhat wanting. This is usually due to the use of an inadequate mold mixture. The following point needs to be understood: it is necessary to get a suitably potent extract to obtain satisfactory results in treatment. Clearly, a good extract (usefulness) depends upon the technique used in growing and harvesting the molds. Homer Prince's study indicated that mold culture broth is by far a larger source of allergen than is the pellicle, which was formerly used for allergen production. The pellicle refers to the mold growth which accumulates in the broth. The MMP (refers to Morrow, Meyer, and Prince, first developers of the method) molds are made from the culture broth and the stock molds from the pellicles alone. During one phase of the clinical investigation conducted in my office, stock molds were used in the treatment of 35 patients who had mold allergy as diagnosed by provocative nasal testing. These patients improved but still had some observable symptoms. These patients were then checked using provocative skin tests, described in a previous chapter. MMP mold extracts were used to determine whether symptoms could be produced in these patients who had been thoroughly treated with the stock molds. Every patient reacted with one or more objective symptoms of congestion, sneezing, coughing, or wheezing. These reactions prove that the protection provided by therapy using the stock molds was insufficient to protect the patient when challenged by provocative skin tests using the MMP molds. All 35 patients who had been on the stock extract were then treated with the MMP extracts. After two to three months of therapy, clinical improvement and even cures invariably resulted!

The preceding example illustrates the necessity of utilizing a highly allergenic mold extract to get good clinical results. Molds made by the MMP process are superior to stock molds when treating allergies. However, sad to say, at the present time, the vast majority of patients suffering from mold allergy are being treated with stock mold extracts rather than by molds made by the MMP process. Thus, it is obvious that the majority of patients suffering from mold allergy are getting ineffectual therapy.

In warm, humid, southeast Texas, molds play an important role in respiratory allergy, but its incidence is approximately 28 per cent in perennial allergy. Yet, figures from various areas of the U. S. show that molds are used in treatment of 65 to 85 per cent of allergic patients. These figures are based upon traditional skin tests and modifications of such tests. This means that approximately 35 to 55 per cent of patients are taking mold shots needlessly!

The percentage of cases who have mold allergy is based upon provocative tests which have a diagnostic efficiency of 90 per cent as indicated in a previous chapter. The diagnostic efficiency of intracutaneous skin tests for molds has a 26 per cent diagnostic efficiency (at best) as indicated previously. Utilizing intracutaneous skin tests for diagnosing mold sensitive patients means that the majority of such patients are receiving treatment which is of no benefit. Also, patients properly diagnosed as having mold allergy but who are being treated with stock molds are getting results which are much less efficient than those treated with molds made by the MMP process. Without question, molds are an important factor in allergy treatment, and leaving out just one mold to which a patient is allergic may yield various degrees of failure.

An interesting side note. There is one particular mold found in moist ground and certain areas of lakes and ponds which might be of significance to a great number of allergy sufferers. That culprit is *Lake Algae*. Subjecting 145 patients with respiratory allergy to *Lake Algae* (using intracutaneous skin tests) yielded 54 positive reactions (35.2 per cent). HOWEVER, PROVOCATIVE NASAL TESTS USING DRIED POWDER OF THIS MOLD YIELDED ONLY 9 POSITIVE TESTS OR ABOUT 6 PER CENT! This illustrates the marked error inherent in the intracutaneous skin testing method. These patients were under specific therapy and all had some degree of trouble with mold allergy. By adding *Lake Algae* to the treatment extract, all 9 patients were markedly improved or cured of their symptoms. The conclusion to be reached from the above example should be clear: allergists must be on the alert for every possible allergen or causative factor in treating patients.

# 11

## *INSECTS IN ALLERGY*

Taking *the sneeze* out of allergies sometimes means focusing on insects as the cause of respiratory allergy. A number of independent studies have shown just that: INSECTS CAN ACT AS AN INHALANT ANTIGEN, THUS CAUSING RESPIRATORY ALLERGIES.

Stevenson and Matthews reported that asthma occurred following provocative bronchial inhalation moth particles. In another case study, two researchers, Feinberg with scratch tests and Wiseman with other skin tests, found a high percentage of positive reactions to insect antigens. Wiseman thought insects might be a significant factor in seasonal respiratory allergy. Van Hoogenhize, using different insects in powdered form and provocative nasal tests, reported positive systemic reactions. In these patients, specific injection therapy brought about clinical improvement.

One hundred and seventy-four respiratory allergy patients were tested at my clinic with intracutaneous skin tests and provocative nasal tests. The common insects, such as crickets, red ants, mosquitoes, spiders, cockroaches, moths, fire ants, and house flies, were dispensed in powdered form for the nasal tests. The standard skin tests were administered using extracts of nine common insects. On the 174 patients administered the skin test, more than half (95), reacted to all nine insect extracts. Twelve per cent (20 patients) reacted to some of the insects, and a third (69) had no reaction at all. Using the provocative nasal test, only a third had positive reactions to ANY of the insects tested, and most of these were from crickets, spiders, red ants, and cockroaches! Then the extremely accurate provocative skin tests were administered to verify the results of the positive nasal tests. These tests showed the nasal tests were only 40 per cent accurate! However, referring to tests for molds and pollens, the provocative skin tests verified results of the nasal tests at an accuracy of 90 per cent.

Interpreting these test results is fairly simple. Comparing numbers of patients who registered positive in the different tests with the numbers who actually were allergic and so verified by provocative testing methods, shows that traditional skin tests are woefully inaccurate. From the above examples, the following fact is inescapable: USING TRADITIONAL SKIN TESTS TO DIAGNOSE INSECT ALLERGIES RESULTED IN 95 PER CENT OF THE PATIENTS RECEIVING USELESS TREATMENT! And that patient who received such treatment as cited above could have been you. Provocative nasal tests can drop that percentage to 60 or less, and provocative skin or eye tests can lower that figure to nearly zero. Provocative eye tests are the method of choice for verifying the nasal tests because, clearly, the provocative skin tests can be, as stated previously, quite traumatic for patients.

The accuracy of testing methods of course varies with the allergen being tested, and so an allergies needs an arsenal of several provocative methods at his disposal to absolutely determine the specific antigen causing the allergy. Also, sniff tests work quite well for evaluating pollens. HOWEVER, THEY WORK

LESS WELL FOR INSECTS, but other techniques can produce results allowing a patient to be free of symptoms in three to five months of treatment. In addition to obvious inherent weaknesses of traditional skin tests, insects, to some extent, undermine *logical method* because they contain histamine which irritates the skin, aside from any allergic considerations. Thus, patients can react to the histamine and not the insect as an allergen! This much is clear: allergists need to properly direct their efforts in treating the patient and his symptoms, not chasing mistaken identities.

# 12

# *HOUSE DUST MITES*

The human being is infested with strange little critters that are, for the most part, not harmful, if such tolerance levels in that particular person are adequate. But, to those who are sensitive to those allergens, watch out! At that point they become a constant source of respiratory allergy. These culprits are microscopic mites that thrive on the dander produced by human skin. The mites are the main element that makes house dust an allergen.

House dust has been recognized as the cause of allergic reactions such as nasal discharge, congestion, post nasal drip, sneezing, hives, coughing or wheezing since the 1920's. However, identifying the specific factor did not occur until the mid '60's when Voorhorst of the Netherlands discovered a correlation between skin tests for house dust and mites.

Controlling the allergy by eliminating the allergen (the *mite)* is not possible because humans carry it with them wherever they go, and it thrives in natural fibers at altitudes under 2,000 feet. The mite population, though, can be reduced by covering cotton mattresses, removing rugs of natural fibers, and, in general, thoroughly cleaning the house. But for respiratory allergy patients to get prime relief (immunization and desensitization) they need allergy shots or injections of mite extract.

The allergenicity of mites and house dust was thoroughly tested at my clinic in the early '70's with provocative skin tests and then compared with traditional skin tests, confirming Voorhorst's results. Six hundred and six patients were tested using provocative skin tests using mite extract, as well as two different dusts from opposing allergy laboratories. The results indicated that the house dust mite was a potent and important allergen for more than half the patients with perennial respiratory allergy. The investigation showed that, while the mite was the most important allergen in house dust, the dust itself also had other allergens of some importance, such as animal dander, insect fragments, molds, pollens, fecal matter, and other materials. These secondary components can be isolated with separate tests to achieve specificity. So, testing dust "by itself" is no longer necessary.

While, generally, traditional intracutaneous tests are poor diagnostic tools, in the case of house dust mites, the tests are about 75 per cent accurate. Remember, though, intracutaneous tests produced poor diagnostic results when used with molds, pollens, and foods. Provocative eye tests, though, effect results that are virtually 100 per cent accurate except for foods. Eye tests, then, are a good way to verify questionable nasal tests results which are still more accurate than traditional scratch and intracutaneous tests. Provocative skin tests are the most accurate, but they can be traumatic for patients without producing, in the case of mites, significantly more accurate results. This is just another indicator that allergists need a wide range of diagnostic tools (and the ability to change such tools based upon the material being tested) to reach an accurate diagnosis AND TO PLAN PROPER TREATMENT.

The provocative nasal test is highly accurate while the ophthalmic or eye test is still as good or better. With these two tests working in tandem at the allergist's command, the correct diagnosis of an inhalant allergy is secure.

This little side note is for those who want to know more about mites. Although there are several types of mites, only two are of clinical importance. One is the American mite (Farinae), the other, European (Pteronyssinus). When the mite was first introduced into the field of allergy, it was thought that the two mites were strikingly similar, and that the American variety was used solely in the U. S. for specific therapy. In later years, this attitude changed, yielding to the idea that, indeed, some minor differences existed. Extracts of both mites were then made for use in the U. S. The two mites were checked with skin tests and yielded different results in specific areas but similar findings overall. Today, extracts are produced for both mites individually and also as a combination.

Not long ago, three patients were treated at my clinic for allergies to the American mite. These patients underwent moderately successful treatment, though it would be stretching the truth to say that such treatment had been a resounding success. The European mite extract was added to the treatment pattern, and within three months all three patients became completely well. Since that time, both types of mite extracts were added to such therapy for anyone suspected of suffering from either mite, and a combined extract of both is now available for mite therapy.

# 13

## *THE SINUSES IN THE FIELD OF ALLERGY*

Four pairs of sinuses are situated in the head: frontal, ethmoid, sphenoid, and maxillary. All the sinuses have openings or *ostia* to permit drainage into the nasal cavity. An infection or allergy may be involved in what is called sinusitis. When this occurs, it is generally assumed to be due to an infection. An x-ray can effectively show the presence of sinusitis but cannot distinguish whether it is due to an allergy, virus, or bacteria. Pain may be experienced when pressure is applied. But, if a patient without sinusitis presses on his face in the sinus areas, he will experience pain. So, in reality, it means nothing. BUT THERE WILL BE evidence of nasal secretions of various degrees and color.

A cytology examination of the secretions from the nasal passages gives a perfect diagnosis of allergy, infection, or both. An infection that is treated with an antibiotic will show a freedom of bacteria within a few days, at which point, the antibiotic can be continued for a period of eight to ten days. If bacteria in some quantity are found after four days of treatment, a culture should be made and sensitivity tests performed to determine the specific antibiotic needed. It should be emphasized here that only one of the sinuses can be affected, or perhaps all eight. But, nevertheless, a MICROSCOPIC EXAMINATION OF NASAL AND BRON-CHIAL SECRETIONS IS NECESSARY FOR PROPER DIAG-NOSIS AND TREATMENT.

Following, are some interesting case studies on this issue. Many years ago a chronic sinusitis patient, Martin Goldman, was referred to my office from another allergist. Mr. Goldman had been suffering from nasal congestion for approximately two years, and past treatment had been ineffective. A cytology examination of the nasal secretions failed to show evidence of infection or allergy. But his history gave evidence of the presence of high blood pressure which was well controlled with medication. A check of the PDR (Physician's Desk Reference) revealed that one of the side effects of the medication in use was nasal congestion! The medication was stopped and a cure followed a week later. A different medication was ordered which gave perfect control of the hypertension without any side effects. Point: a simple cytology examination led to a quick cure which was not only satisfying but of very minor expense.

Another case involved a man from Port Arthur, Texas, Jonathan Lynch, with severe, killing-type headaches. This particular case goes back some 40 years. An immediate x-ray of the sinuses had been made which showed a marked sinusitis in only one sinus, namely the right sphenoid sinus. We decided to call in a very excellent Ear, Nose, and Throat (ENT) specialist and asked him to wash out the sinus and please send a sample of the washings. Almost immediately, relief followed the sinus irrigation. A micro-scopic examination of the secretions revealed 4-Plus Eosinophiles and no bacteria. This indicated a simple allergy. Mr. Lynch was very allergic to house dust, and rapid immunization was begun. Two more sinus irritations became necessary in the following weeks, with relief following thereafter. Immunization continued for a few weeks. Later, Mr. Lynch took early retirement due to a heart condition, but the sinus allergy remained in complete control. During this retirement period, Mr. Lynch often went hunting in the woods near his town. One day when he failed to return home on schedule, his wife went to his favorite hunting area, which she knew well, and found him slumped against a tree, dead for a number of hours. In his lap was an open bottle of pills to be used in case of a heart attack. Even though other bodily functions, in My Lynch's case totally unrelated to allergy, are not in good working order, proper provocative diagnosis can still lead to a total cure.

A middle-aged woman, Ann Jeffries, from Houston, Texas, had been referred to my office in the late '70's, suffering from frequent headaches and mild nasal symptoms of a few year's duration. A microscopic examination of Ann's nasal secretions revealed the presence of eosinophiles which was diagnostic of allergy (evidence that the headaches were associated with nasal allergy). Foods and inhalants proved negative, and pointed to the possible and probable that her allergy was triggered by her surroundings. When she left home for several hours at a time to go most anywhere, she would virtually clear up completely. She also would frequently drive a long distance to visit a distant shopping center, and she would remain free of symptoms only as long as she stayed away from four particular stores. When she didn't, she would return home and her headaches and nasal congestion were already blooming in full force. It was discovered that her bedroom, where she spent a good part of the day, was situated over the garage where her teenage son spent long hours most everyday working on his car and various household appliances. By observation, Ann found that in the shopping center there were four stores that she usually frequented, and usually on the same trip, stores that had strong perfume and new clothes odors. The garage at home also had similar odor types and was shut down and the garage material moved to another site. A special rubber mask with filters was fitted, to be worn by Ann when visiting the specific four stores in the shopping center. This simple procedure yielded complete freedom from her symptoms. In this case, creative detective work by the patient paid off in big dividends.

Another interesting case study involved Robert Simmons of Little Rock, Arkansas, a 35-year-old junior college teacher who complained of headaches for a year or more. Robert's symptoms seemed to emanate from the area in which he lived. His home was in the country and surrounded by pine trees, resulting in air that also contained the pleasant odor of pine. When he occasionally left the area, overnight, his headaches would leave. This was an obvious case of pine odor sensitivity. An extract of pine odor was made for therapy. This was done by using a De Vilbus pump which generated a bottle of extracting fluid. The odorous air was pumped into the bottle all night for two nights. An extract of this pine odor was made in my laboratory and used in a program of desensitization. Within four months, complete desensitization occurred which led to a complete remission of symptoms. Another similar case was treated the same way, but the medication used was made by the extraction of the pine element from pine cones.

# 14

## *PRESERVATIVES IN FOOD*

Since the beginning of time, allergy has been associated with dust, molds, pollens, animal dander, and man's survival sustenance, FOOD. We now know that chemicals in our food supply as well as in the air play a significant role in our physical and mental well being.

*Sulphite* chemicals are particularly to blame, the critters used to keep food fresh and attractive in appearance. These *sulphites* are used in many processed foods including fruit drinks, beer, wine, baked goods, dried fruit and vegetables, and in the processing of some food ingredients including gelatin, beet sugar, corn sweeteners, and food starches.

Since 1959, six *sulphite* agents have been listed as "generally recognized" as safe for food use. These agents are *sulphur dioxide, sodium sulphite, sodium and potassium bisulphite, and sodium and potassium metabisulphite.* Testing for allergy reactions to the chemical *sulphite* produced interesting results. My clinic conducted an investigation of 200 patients with general allergies consisting of asthma, nasal allergy, headaches and other related symptoms. Two capsules containing a total of 1,000 mg (1/4 teaspoon) of *sodium bisulphite and sodium metabisulphite* were swallowed on an empty stomach with 30 minutes allowed to elapse for a reaction to occur. Twenty patients (ten per cent) reacted with attacks of asthma, nasal allergy, headaches, gastrointestinal symptoms or a combination of such problems. In all cases, patient suffering was relieved by an injection of adrenalin (a medication used to abort allergy attacks).

Tammy Smith, a 14-year-old student-athlete from Houston, Texas, came to my office with a history of frequent hospitalizations. For years, she had been treated by doctors employing traditional allergy methods, and, at the time I first saw her, she was as "successfully healed" by these methods as she was going to get, to the extent that she only had mild to moderate attacks of asthma and nasal allergy, controllable with home medication. Digging deeper into her problem, we discovered that most of her attacks occurred after school. During this late afternoon time period, she almost daily ate a hamburger and french fries. Suspecting the agent *sulphite as* the problem, we subjected Tammy to an oral challenge of *sulphite* capsules. Within 15 minutes, she began to sneeze, cough, and wheeze! This was the answer! The culprit of her persistent asthma and nasal allergy was the french fries which she ate almost daily! Elimination of the french fries from Tammy's diet led to freedom from her trouble. Remember: all french fries contain the *sulphite* chemical which keeps this appealing food fresh in appearance!

John Mark, a 40-year-old bricklayer in San Antonio, Texas, came to see me one day, suffering from chronic asthma. At the time, he was under treatment with another doctor, but he came to my clinic because we had successfully treated a friend of his some months before. John frequently had mild wheezing under the medication he was taking at the time, but it was not an incapacitating condition. Still, he was bothered enough to investigate if there was anything we could do for him. A challenge test with *sulphites* produced asthma within 20 minutes! Do you have any idea what solved his problem? Let me drop a hint here. It has to do with liquid intake. Got it yet? John was cured of all wheezing when he stopped drinking three bottles of beer a day! All beer contains the *sulphite* chemical, and no amount of preventive medication can completely eliminate the unwanted side effects (wheezing, etc.) *of sulphite* intake for the unwary sufferer. These two case studies adequately illustrate the problems some people have with the *sulphite* chemical. However, *sulphite* alone is not the only problem.

Let's take a look at another "highwayman" that can make your life miserable if you are a person who suffers from its ingestion and likes food that contains the culprit agent. No medical study is complete without taking a look at *monosodium glutamate,* used in some processed foods and especially in a number of sausages and lunch meats. In the summer of 1981, 100 allergy patients were tested at my clinic by oral challenge with *monosodium glutamate.* Five patients reacted with either asthma, nasal allergy, headaches, gastrointestinal symptoms, or a combination of problems. In one patient, Mary Adams, an executive secretary from Durant, Oklahoma, *monosodium glutamate* was the sole cause of her chronic headaches! Simply by reading labels on processed foods, Mary easily eliminated those foods containing the cause of her problem. As a result, her headache malady was solved.

Another important culprit to be aware of is *sodium nitrite.* This chemical is found in almost all bacon, lunch meats, sausages, and hams. A little side note: Owens Sausage does not use *sodium nitrite* in its products but does use *monosodium glutamate* as a preservative. Also, in some other brands of sausage, both *sodium nitrite and monosodium glutamate* are used.

*Sodium nitrite* came to my interest because of its frequent use in packaged meats. Upon researching existing literature on *sodium nitrite,* no reference to this chemical was found as a causative factor or allergen in cases of allergy. Using capsules containing 50 mg of *sodium nitrite* (1/80th teaspoon) an investigation of 100 patients was conducted at my clinic. Patient symptoms ranged from asthma, nasal allergy, headaches, gastrointestinal problems, to various combinations. The test dosage was 50 mg of *sodium nitrite,* about the same amount as found in one pound of preserved meat. Sixteen of the 100 patients severely reacted to the *sodium nitrite* injection, and ALL 16 PATIENTS cleared up immediately (within 15 minutes) after receiving injections of adrenalin! Contrary to popular opinion even within medical circles, *sodium nitrite* is a triggering device to allergic reactions in patients susceptible to this chemical.

The next case study is specifically mentioned for headache sufferers, and *sodium nitrite* is still on the hook. Evelyn Jones, a 40-year-old wife of a Baptist minister in Lubbock, Texas, had severe and frequent headaches when she came to my office in early 1981. An allergic factor was suspected because all past treatments she had received elsewhere had failed to bring relief. Upon subjecting Evelyn to a complete allergy panel, no evidence indicated anything adverse to food or inhalant allergies. At this time, it just so happened my office was investigating *sodium nitrite* as an allergen and, as such, Evelyn was included within the study. She reacted with a very severe headache within 20 minutes following injection, which was relieved by an injection of adrenalin. If Evelyn had come to my office just a month before, sorry to say, we would have failed to find the *etiologic* factor causing her problem. How many cases in the past that slipped through undetected is inestimable. Evelyn's problem was correctly isolated and solved. Point: the patient needs to be tested for all possible solutions, including *sodium nitrite.*

One last case study while we are on this subject. Forty-five-year-old Jenny James, a computer scientist with a large firm in the Dallas area, came to my office as an on-then-off sufferer from intestinal problems, possibly allergy related. The word "possibly" is used in the above thought because a year previously Jenny's symptoms had cleared up on an elimination diet, but challenge feeding proved negative. The reason for this is because only untreated foods are used in such challenges. Jenny was seen at my office at the time of the *sulphite* investigations, and it was learned that she habitually ate bacon for breakfast, lunch meat for lunch, and ham or sausage about three times a week for supper. Jenny was put on a meat-free diet. She returned in four days completely free of intestinal symptoms. At that point, free of the allergen within her system causing the problem, a capsule containing 50 mg of *sodium nitrite* was administered on an empty stomach. Within 25 minutes, she reacted with all the usual intestinal symptoms! In the majority of allergy cases, quite frequently, multiple *etiological* factors surface, but not infrequently only one factor may stand out as the sole causative agent. In this case, the elimination of *sodium nitrite* yielded a clinical cure in Jenny's case.

A few thoughts are presented here to wind up this chapter and tie things together. In the sulphite investigation, 16 per cent of allergic patients had a diagnostic reaction. Think of 1,000 or even 100,000 or more people with hidden allergies who, everyday, react to this commonly used chemical in our food supply! Hundreds of thousands of people with common allergies are getting treatment with little or only partial improvement because one factor is overlooked.

At the present time, a very minor number of patients with multiple allergies are being tested for *sodium nitrite or* other preservatives which may well rest upon *etiological* factors. Let's be reasonable: any person can do this test by eliminating meat intake containing *sodium nitrite*. If that person is then well or markedly improved, just add such foods to the diet and watch for reactions. It is not any more complicated than that! Still better, if your doctor will administer a capsule containing 50 mg of this chemical on an empty stomach, you will have a reaction (if so affected) and thus produce an accurate diagnosis within 30 minutes. And, of course, an injection of adrenalin will stop the reaction within minutes.

# 15

# *HOUSE DUST IN THE FIELD OF ALLERGY*

In approximately 1920, house dust was introduced as an allergen thought to cause respiratory allergy, especially bronchial asthma. However, the use of house dust in therapy gave variable results. Skin tests, especially the intracutaneous tests, were frequently positive. Clinical results followed in various degrees of success due to the contents of different dusts produced. Dust was gathered in homes from mattresses, rugs, carpets, window sills, closets and every other source-producing area. Every batch of dust collected varied in contents and, after extraction, the extracts varied in specificity. In addition to the unknown factors in these *dusts* were insects, molds, pollens, animal dander, and who knows what else.

In 1930, Dr. Bernard Efron, an excellent allergist of the day and a good researcher, theorized that the essential allergen in house dust came from the breakdown products of aging cotton. In that era, all mattresses were made of cotton. He believed that if you collected a

64

pound of cotton from the fields, sterilized the cotton, then placed the contents in a jar to age in a refrigerator for a year, this *clean cotton* would contain the true allergen or antigen of house dust. This was a theory which Efron never put into practice.

What did happen was that Efron made his house dust from old cotton mattresses only and thus got a superior and effective dust. Over the years it proved a very successful dust in the practice of allergy. Since I had a close association with Dr. Efron, I had an ample source of this potent house dust extract which gave me the edge in the practice of allergy.

As you might expect, each batch of dust contained a mixture of antigens, and each batch varied in consistency. If a new batch was introduced for therapy, it was essential to go back one dilution to prevent overdosing. Explanation: if a patient was on a dilution of 1:100, the next starting dose from a new batch of extract was set at 1:1000. The clinical results using Efron's dust proved much superior to dust used in those cases using a less perfect dust extract. After several years of clinical use, a good market within the field of allergy was generated for Dr. Efron's dust, and Endo laboratories then produced the dust for general use.

In the early 1970's, I did provocative skin tests using Endo dust and found it very effective with a high diagnostic efficiency of 75 per cent or better. However, two years later, this previously excellent dust proved ineffective for use in therapy. I then redid my previous study using provocative skin testing. This investigation proved that the Endo dust of two years previously was of little value. Correspondence with Endo regarding my findings was initiated. Endo wrote back and said that the old cotton mattresses obtained from mattress companies had been depleted and that, in large part, plastic had been substituted.

Endo laboratories responded by obtaining cotton from the fields and aging the material for 18 months then making the previously superior dust from the aged cotton. The answer was still missing, and Endo took the dust off the market.

At this particular time, mites were discovered. It was the mites in house dust which supplied the principle allergenic factor. Since mites were carried on the skin, they easily fell off and found a new home in the mattresses, thus thriving on the cotton from which the mattresses were made!

However, let's be clear on this point. The house dust principle is still used by many allergists along with mite extract. This is needless. Other ingredients in house dust should be individually checked for and used as necessary in therapy. To get the best results, we need to follow the rule of specificity and not treat the patient only in general terms.

# 16

# *RESPIRATORY ALLERGY AND INFECTION*

A widely held opinion suggests that respiratory allergy is related to respiratory infection, especially in children under the age of ten and in adults over 40. Because of this opinion, much effort has been spent trying to prevent infection as a means of controlling bronchial and nasal allergy, including bronchial asthma.

Gallons of vaccines, some made from the patient's own germs, others mixed from stock supplies, have been used for years with conflicting results. Personally, I used such vaccines for my first 20 years in clinical allergy and thought they helped patients, but, over the past 30 years of using provocative allergy tests, I realized that the vaccine therapy principle did little or nothing to end the allergic illness in patients.

Respiratory tract infections may be viral or bacterial in origin. These infections may or may not be accompanied by fever, low or high blood counts. The presence of infection can be determined by testing for bacteria in the respiratory tract. Normal nasal cavities, sinuses, and the bronchial tree are usually free of bacteria or germs which normally exist in the nasopharynx (rear area of the nasal passages). When antibacterial barriers are broken by lowered resistance of the nasal mucous lining, nasopharynx bacteria spreads into the normally germ-free areas.

Although the respiratory tract has many openings that provide easy access for bacteria, the body generally protects itself. The mouth and nasal openings continually secrete mucous that is swallowed, sweeping the bacteria to the stomach where the germs are digested. Saliva offers additional protection with its antibiotic action. The few bacteria that do reach the lungs are likely trapped in mucous and then kicked out by the sweeping action of tiny hairs called ciliary cells that line the respiratory passages. Once bacteria are swept to the esophagus, the unwanted intruders are swallowed and digested.

Microscopic examination of nasal secretions from the upper and lower respiratory tract can determine with great statistical accuracy the presence of viral or bacterial infections. The color or amount of secretions does not necessarily indicate infection. The color depends on the number of cells in the mucous, not on the presence or absence of infection. But the microscopic examination of secretions is 90 per cent accurate in determining the presence of infection.

*The respiratory tract* includes every area from the nasal openings down through the bronchial tubes to the lung air sacs. The linings or mucous membranes of these areas are similar in structure. An infection or allergy may start in the nose and remain there, or it may be continuous through the bronchial area down to the lung air sacs.

The microscopic examination of secretions is a quick and inexpensive way to determine whether allergy, infection, or both exist. If the examination shows neutrophiles (blood cells that fight infection) and bacteria, then clearly an infection is present. When eosinophiles (blood cells that fight allergy) are present, the cause of symptoms is allergy. When a combination of neutrophiles, bacteria, and eosinophiles are present, infection and allergy are involved. Use of antibiotics eliminate the bacteria, and lack of bacteria in the secretions indicate the infection has cleared. If the symptoms also clear, then the infection was the cause. If symptoms persist and eosinophiles are present, then, allergy, not infection was the cause of illness.

Based upon microscopic studies of respiratory secretions in 375 cases of bronchial asthma without fever, infection was found in 109 cases, or 28.3 per cent. The remaining 267, or 71.7 per cent, were free of infection. The breakdown of infection by age group was: patients under the age of three, 31.2 per cent; from age three to twelve, 30.4 per cent; 12 to 40, 10.1 per cent; and 40 years of age and older, 28.3 per cent.

A second series of 202 cases involving asthmatic bronchitis showed essentially the same associated rate of infection as those cases with bronchial asthma. Asthmatic bronchitis refers to an inflammation of the bronchial tubes accompanied by coughing but little or no wheezing or shortness of breath. Bronchial asthma refers to a bronchial muscle spasm resulting in wheezing and shortness of breath.

THE ISSUE OF TREATING INFECTIONS WITH ANTIBIOTICS IS IMPORTANT. In children under the age of three, test results showed that eliminating the infection is of clinical importance. However, in patients over three, the use of antibiotics results in little significant change in the asthmatic state. In none of these cases could germs or bacteria be cited as the specific cause of the allergic condition.

Due to the similarity of findings in bronchial asthma and asthmatic bronchitis, the following study results are enlightening. In

148 cases with fever, 73 or 48.2 per cent involved infection. In the age group up to three years, the incidence was 41.2 per cent; three to twelve, 42.2 per cent; and 12 to 40 years, 16.6 per cent.

No correlation between asthma and respiratory infection was found. That is, no significant relationship existed between the onset of asthma and fever. More frequently, the fever seemed to follow the onset of asthma.

In cases of bronchial asthma with fever but without infection, shown by the absence of germs or bacteria, the chief finding is dehydration, as plugs of secretion block one or more areas of the bronchial tubes, thus initiating fever. If this condition is not remedied, infection invariably follows. Patients with plugged bronchial tubes are treated symptomatically, usually with intravenous fluids containing antispasmodics. Generally, such treatment relieves asthmatic symptoms, the fever disappearing within 24 hours.

The case of six-year-old Rodney Jones of El Paso, Texas, illustrates a key point. He came to us with a temperature of 103 with respiratory infection associated with a heavy cough and some mild shortness of breath. The examination revealed pneumonia in the lower right lung. The cytology examination of coughed-up secretions showed a marked presence of eosinophiles which denoted allergy. Bacteria were absent which was evidence of no infection. A diagnosis of bronchial asthma was made with dehydration and blocking of the bronchial tubes of the right lung. An infusion of fluids was initiated in the vein with aminphylum in the fluids. This medication was used to dilate and relieve the asthmatic spasms of the bronchial tubes. Fluids were given over a period of three hours. At this time, the child began to cough and suddenly a gush of thick secretions were expelled. A microscopic analysis again showed only eosinophiles and no bacteria. The examination showed relief of the bronchial obstruction of the right lung. Antibiotics were not prescribed. The child had a good night sleep and woke up in the morning free of fever and breathing was normal, and he went to school that morning.

Many children under the age of three years have frequent respiratory tract infections because of immature lymphocytic systems. Their bodies do not develop adequate immunity against infection. By the age of four years, these children develop mature lymphocytes and stop having such infections.

Many pediatric allergists predict that these frequent infections eventually lead to bronchial asthma. Therefore, these allergists advise allergic testing and therapy at an early age as a means of preventing future allergic states. As a pediatrician and allergist, I have seen far too many infants and children in this age bracket survive bouts with "colds" without harm. The repeated infections suddenly cease once the youngsters reach age four, or so, and this "outgrowing" of "colds" comes about without subjecting the children to therapeutic treatment.

Far too many infants and children undergo skin testing and then take "shots" for three years or more for their so-called allergic conditions. Key point: children who start with allergy injections at three to eleven months clear up wonderfully well at three to four years of age, JUST LIKE THOSE CHILDREN WHO ARE NOT SUBJECTED TO SUCH THERAPY! Often, the treatment for these children are injections for dust, molds, and pollens based upon traditional skin tests. These tests are basically inaccurate and their value even more diminished in infancy and childhood.

While many children and older age groups "outgrow" their allergies, this does not mean these patients should be neglected and specific therapy left out. Not at all. But clinical results (relief of symptoms) should be readily apparent in the majority of cases in three to five months of treatment initiation.

As for "outgrowing" allergies, reference is made to Buffum and Assettipone who reported on 518 asthma patients who had no specific treatment. Ten years after the first visit to a treatment center, 41 per cent were free of symptoms; 52.4 per cent had only slight or occasional asthmatic symptoms; and 6.6 per cent still had enough asthma to be handicapped.

Moreover, Johnstone investigated 91 children with asthma four years after their initial visit to an allergist. The study showed that 18 per cent were free of asthma; and 22.2 per cent were free of asthma by 16 years of age. Furthermore, Montgomery and Smith showed that 75 per cent of 95 children with asthma had less trouble five years later while 30 per cent had not had an attack in the last year of the study.

Clearly, infants and small children who have frequent colds are not necessarily allergic nor are they destined to remain victims of allergy. The blind handling of these children as allergic sufferers with the resulting use of skin tests and injection therapy is without foundation or benefit. The same results can be obtained through benign neglect without the trauma and needless expense of so-called "skin tests" and "shots."

# 17

# *SECRETORY OTITIS MEDIA*

Ringing in the ear or *tinnitus* along with other middle ear problems may be related to nasal allergy. Other symptoms may include a feeling of fullness, stuffiness, or pressure in the ear. Hearing problems may be present ranging from almost insignificant to complete deafness. Patients may complain of a sensation like water bubbling in the ear. Younger children and infants may never complain and the ailment goes unnoticed for weeks or months until progressive deafness causes the youngsters to become inattentive. Infants and children under four years of age may show signs or restlessness and pull at the affected ear.

The relationship of allergy and diseases of the middle *ear, secretory otitis media,* caught my attention in 1959, and I first wrote about it then. Problems of the middle ear generally occur because the eustachian tube (tube connecting the middle ear with the pharynx or throat) cannot function properly. This tube normally performs an aeration function. When that function is interrupted, it leads to absorption of air in the middle ear. This process causes a vacuum which draws fluid into the middle ear. Or an inflammation of the tube may produce a fluid, again, filling the middle ear or tympanic cavity with fluid. Generally, the fluid in both cases is sterile, and the ailment is called *secretory otitis media*. This diagnosis can be easily reached through a routine eardrum examination (ear drum doesn't look normal).

Eustachian tube blockage has a number of causes which may produce swelling of the tube lining or closure of the tube opening. Such conditions are acute upper respiratory infection, acute and chronic sinusitis, chronic nasopharyngitis, and nasal allergy.

Compression or closure of the tube may also be caused by tumors in the back, nasal part of the throat, or by enlarged adenoids. Interference in the normal tubal function occurs when there are rapid changes in pressure on the other side of the eardrum as in rapid descent in an airplane or elevator. Infection is the most common cause of tube swelling with the resulting middle ear fluid problem. Nasal allergy plays a minor but significant role in tubal swelling.

Excessively large adenoids are the most common cause of compression or closure of the tube. The trigger mechanism may be infection, allergy, or a combination of the two. Allergy and infection may cause the adenoids to swell which may be just enough to complete closure of the tube. When the adenoids are removed, the tube may remain open just long enough to avoid the middle ear problem regardless of repeated allergic or infectious flare-ups.

The biggest cause of middle ear problems as a chronic ailment is failure on the part of the doctor to do microscopic and cultural tests for bacterial infection. These doctors all too often rely upon clinical evidence of improvement which causes too many residual infections to go untreated. Also, doctors often fail to recognize the presence of allergy, alone or in combination with infection.

Treatment of *secretory otitis media* should be directed at eliminating swelling of the eustachian tube lining. With swelling not a problem, the tube will open and normal functions will be restored. In a few cases, the fluid may have become gelatinous with the possible formation of scar tissue which requires the eardrum to be surgically opened so the middle ear cavity can be cleared of the material. Such surgery, however, should be used as a last resort.

The popular treatment of this middle ear disorder involves introduction of a polyethylene tube through the eardrum into the middle ear which provides instant relief. The tube may stay in place anywhere from three to twenty-four months and then fall out. As long as the plastic tube is in place, the problem will not reoccur.

Personally, I do not recommend use of the tube in the early stages of ailment. The first step should be diagnosing and eliminating the cause of the problem, if possible. If, after diligent investigation and therapy, there is no relief or there are frequent recurrences, the use of the plastic tube is indicated.

A key tool for determining the presence of allergy or infection involves the microscopic examination of nasal secretions. Normal nasal cavities, sinuses, and bronchial tree are free of germs. If nasal cavity secretions show microscopic evidence of bacteria and neutrophiles (blood cells that fight infections), then a diagnosis of infection can be made. If eosinophiles are present, then an allergy is the cause. Of course, all three may be present, meaning allergy and infection are involved.

Antibiotics can clear the infection, but it is important to retest for bacteria even though the patient is better. It is persistent infection in the face of clinical results that accounts for the persistence of eustachian tube swelling and retention of fluid in the middle ear. If bacteria are still present, a sensitivity test must be done to determine the specific antibiotic needed. Allergic therapy should involve ACIH and Prednisolone (a Cortisone analogue). Antihistamines can be used, but will not by themselves lead to a clinical cure. If symptoms persist, then use of the polyethylene tube is indicated.

Too many children receive needless treatment because their ailment is routinely misdiagnosed as allergic in nature. Doctors insert tubes in the youngsters' ears, perform skin tests, and begin injection therapy for things ranging from dust, molds, and pollens. Between the tubes and allergy shots, these children for the most part get well in time, but not because of the allergy routine. The shape of the eustachian tube in children under the age of eight, and even more so under the age of six, predisposes it to the middle ear ailment. As the child gets older, the tube is gradually converted from the easily infected childhood type to the adult type which is much less susceptible to infection.

The real answer to the issue of clinical cures is the anatomical change along with the development of a more mature immunological system which reduces risk of infections. Success is not the blind use of injections of multiple antigens by traditional allergists that results in "cures."

# 18

## *BRONCHIAL ASTHMA*

Asthma can be a debilitating ailment. Its causes are frequently misdiagnosed and obvious allergic ties often overlooked. Bronchial asthma refers to a wheezing type of breathing that is especially evident during a long exhalation of breath. It is produced by a constriction or narrowing of the air passages in the lungs. This constriction may be due to a spasm of the bronchial muscles, swelling of the mucous membrane lining, or thickened mucous plugs or a combination of all three.

Causes of these reactions are usually classified into four categories: factors outside the body; factors operating inside the body; allergic conditions; and things nonallergic. Allergic asthma is the description used when the condition is accompanied by positive skin tests for allergies. With nonallergic asthma, there are no positive skin tests.

Skin tests, though, are a poor criteria for determining the causes of an allergic reaction because of their inherent inaccuracies. As for wheezing, the old axiom, *all is not asthma that wheezes,* holds true. Any obstruction of the bronchi or airways, such as foreign bodies or growths, will cause wheezing. Wheezing also may occur with chronic bronchitis, pneumoconiosis (miner's lung), and cardiac failure. These conditions are serious and must be ruled out, but the possibility of an allergic condition should not be overlooked.

The term "asthma" can be applied or misapplied to a variety of conditions and is better understood by looking at bronchial asthma versus asthmatic bronchitis. *Bronchial asthma* includes spasms of the bronchial muscles accompanied by a shortness of breath. The symptoms can be dramatically relieved by bronchial dilators such as Adrenalin or Aminophyllin. *Asthmatic bronchitis* results in little or no shortness of breath. It does not respond to the drugs that relieve bronchial asthma. This condition often includes a cough, with or without mild wheezing or bronchial discomfort and other subjective symptoms.

My experience indicates there is no reason to classify respiratory allergy as resulting from factors inside or outside the body, allergic or nonallergic. Asthma is asthma, and there is an identifiable cause, although that cause may be elusive in many cases. The failure to diagnose the factors causing the asthma is no reason to call it intrinsic. Nor is the absence of positive skin tests a reason to view nonallergic asthma as an ailment unto itself

Far too many cases of emphysema, chronic bronchitis, and bronchial asthma are lumped together or diagnostically thrown in a convenient wastebasket because of the improper or inadequate use of available diagnostic tools for determining the causes of allergy. Traditional allergists still rely on voluminous histories and skin tests for diagnosis, but these methods rarely give complete or partially complete answers.

Even with emphysema and all the suffering it entails, allergy can be a complicating factor in a large percentage of cases. Controlling the allergy often reverses or relieves many of the symptoms. Bronchial asthma, classic in the way its symptoms present themselves, is easily recognized as an allergic condition by the doctor and patient. However, it is not as easy to identify the allergic basis for patients with bronchitis and emphysema and the corresponding coughing, phlegm, and lack of wheezing. Confirmation of allergy's role is need enough for these cases which typically occur in people over 50 years of age.

Microscopic examination of the phlegm or secretions can yield special insight as to whether the ailment is allergic. The presence of eosinophilia suggests allergy as the cause. Bacteria suggest infection. Both may be present. A course of the proper antibiotic should relieve symptoms in four or five days, if the symptoms are caused by the infection. A second microscopic examination is important to check for bacteria and eosinophilia (continued presence of bacteria indicates the proper antibiotic was not used). Once the bacteria are eliminated, patients may experience some relief, but the continued presence of eosinophilia means the ailment is allergy related.

Janice Barnes, a 65-year-old secretary with a large law firm in Austin, came to us with severe emphysema. She was dyspneic, malnourished with severe swelling of the feet and ankles. She spent 24 hours a day in a wheelchair, as she could not breathe lying down. Her lungs were clear with distant breath sounds. Bronchial secretions were free of bacteria but presented a marked eosinophilia, indicating a true allergic condition with markedly advanced emphysema. Janice was examined and all tests for inhalants like dust and molds were negative. She was then hospitalized and placed on a therapeutic fast. She had to sit up in bed and was supported by pillows. Under these severe conditions, she remarked that all she wanted in life was to be able to lay down in bed at night and to have the ability to walk across the room. I promised her just that.

After three full days of fasting and an adequate intake of spring water, she could lay down on her back without pillows to prop her up! I'll never forget that particular day. When I walked into her hospital room during my morning rounds, she beamed ear to ear when she saw me, and said, "Leave me be, doctor. I'm living it up!"

On the food challenge, Janice was found to be allergic to five commonly eaten foods. She was discharged shortly thereafter and was instructed to completely avoid those foods. She lived comfortably free of her former condition until she died suddenly from heart failure about a year later.

For those over 50 years old, other considerations enter into the picture. Allergy that occurs in patients of this age bracket may be complicated in chronic, recurrent infections, but they are, nonetheless, basically allergic in nature. The proper control of the allergy generally controls recurrent infections, but these cases seldom show positive skin tests and are of little diagnostic significance. Most of these patients have food sensitivities as the major cause of symptoms (Chapter 19).

Inhalants may play a significant role in some asthma cases occurring in older people. Inhalants can best be diagnosed by provocative nasal and eye tests. These patients often have an accompanying sinus allergy that includes symptoms such as post nasal drip, some degree of nasal congestion and throat-clearing after meals.

Food challenges produce striking results. Sam Turner, a 70-year-old man and a former high-rise welder, came to see me in the late '70's with severe emphysema and spent his days in a rocking chair on his front porch. Sam had a tank of oxygen at his side which he used for prolonged intervals during the day. Bronchial secretions showed a predominance of eosinophiles, indicating the presence of an associated allergy along with advanced emphysema. Hospitalization was ordered, and Sam was put on a therapeutic fast. In four days, Sam was breathing with little difficulty, with loss of coughing and a greatly increased sense of well being. Food challenges indicated that he was allergic to five common foods. He left the hospital and returned to the chair on his front porch but without the oxygen tank!

# 19

## FOOD ALLERGY

Foods are of great importance in the field of allergy, serving as a prominent offender in 75 per cent of perennial allergy patients! After testing 1,000 patients under hospital controlled conditions, it was found that foods alone were involved in 50 per cent of the cases, with inhalants the offending agent 25 per cent of the time!

Dr. Theron Randolph of Chicago, one of the first allergists to recognize the importance of foods in allergy, agrees on the role foods play in clinical allergy. But not all allergists agree! In fact, allergists at one national meeting, while agreeing that foods played a role in allergy, varied on the scope of that role from five to seventy-five percent! When seasoned allergists voice such differences of opinion, little can be said for the stability of this specialty as practiced by traditional allergists using traditional testing methods.

The vast difference of opinion is due to the varied and uncontrolled methods of arriving at a diagnosis of food allergy. Skin tests are used by the majority of clinical allergists, and, yet, the diagnostic efficiency of skin tests is quite low. Many allergists rely on a patient's history to diagnose food allergy, but such a history is of dubious value. It is a rare patient who can identify the foods that cause his symptoms, and, anyway, most patients deny that foods cause allergy symptoms. Patients who do recognize foods as causing some symptoms cannot, of course, identify all the foods involved.

A variety of elimination diets have been used as a way of diagnosing which foods cause adverse reactions. One method advocates fasting a patient for one to three days, then adding a new food every two or three days to see if a reaction occurs. This is commonly referred to as *challenge feeding*. The problem with this diet alone is that a patient is rarely clear of all symptoms in one to three days. Adding a new food to the patient's diet who is not completely free of symptoms leads to multiple errors.

Another popular method is to place a patient for two weeks on a diet consisting of 20 to 30 foods that supposedly are infrequent causes of trouble for most people. Then, the so called allergenic foods, or foods considered common causes of allergy, are added to the diet, one at a time every one to three days. The problem here is that the foods seldom causing problems are main offenders.

Cereal free and fruit-free diets have many advocates, but I have yet to see a patient in whom cereals and fruits were the only offenders. Quite simply, all foods or additives are potentially suspect. Some allergists recommend eliminating all foods in the same biological family (guilt by association), but the practice is unjustified. Foods in the same family may have some common similarities or antigens, but there is not enough of a relationship to justify eliminating several related foods. For example, tomato, potato, and tobacco are in the same family, but the odds of all three causing trouble in the same patient are remote. Point: NO MATTER WHAT ELIMINATION DIET IS USED, THE PATIENT MUST BE COMPLETELY OR ALMOST COMPLETELY FREE

OF ALL SYMPTOMS AT THE TIME HE IS CHALLENGED
WITH THE FOOD BEING TESTED.

In tests of 50 consecutive allergy patients at my clinic in the
early '70's, it was found that the average patient was allergic to
nine foods based on trial feedings, those completely free of symptoms at the time of challenge. The patients were then challenged
with 40 foods, food additives, or condiments. Of the 50 patients,
fewer than five were allergic to the same foods.

The foods and condiments tested were: wheat, milk, egg, beef,
pork, potato, coffee, chocolate, rice, black pepper, red pepper,
chicken, orange, tomato, cane sugar, Brewer's yeast, Baker's yeast,
string beans, peanuts, lettuce, corn, tobacco, onion, celery, green
pepper, tea, garlic, mustard, malt, vanilla, cinnamon, oats, lemon,
fish, shellfish, food color, caramel, soybeans, sunflower oil, and
cottonseed oil.

To show the diversity of specific foods causing allergic symptoms, 50 consecutive patients with food allergies were given the
foods responsible for their symptoms. Patients experienced reactions from one to twenty-five foods. The average number in this
series was 9.2. The following table illustrates the challenge concept using 38 common foods.

A considerable number of foods causing specific symptoms
in the patients used for compiling figures for the following tables
are among the foods generally considered by traditional allergists
as "safe" or having little importance in causing allergic reactions.
As I have said previously, the most important foods in allergy
are those that cause specific reactions for you, and that means all
foods are under suspicion. The 38 foods and condiments used in
the following provocative tests all gave reactions rating in
importance from a low of 4 per cent to a high of 40 per cent.

Once a patient knows his sensitivity to the 38 foods, he can
begin testing the other foods he eats frequently. The patient can
follow the same routine used in testing the above foods to determine

## REACTIONS TO FOODS IN 50 CONSECUTIVE PATIENTS WITH FOOD ALLERGY (1)

| Foods | Reaction Number | Foods | Reaction Number |
|---|---|---|---|
| Baker's Yeast | 16 | Milk | 17 |
| Beef | 18 | Malt | 10 |
| Brewer's Yeast | 12 | Onion | 14 |
| Black Pepper | 11 | Orange | 16 |
| Chicken | 13 | Peanut | 13 |
| Coffee | 13 | Potato | 7 |
| Cotton | 13 | Pork | 13 |
| Caramel | 9 | Rice | 5 |
| Celery | 10 | Red Pepepr | 12 |
| Celery | 10 | Sugar | 8 |

## REACTIONS TO FOODS IN 50 CONSECUTIVE PATIENTS WITH FOOD ALLERGY (2)

| Foods | Reaction Number | Foods | Reaction Number |
|---|---|---|---|
| Chocolate | 20 | Shell Fish | 14 |
| Cinnamon | 10 | St. Beans | 2 |
| Corn | 19 | Soybeans | 5 |
| Egg | 19 | Safflower Oil | 8 |
| Fish | 12 | Tobacco | 8 |
| Food Color | 11 | Tea | 11 |
| Green Pepper | 12 | Tomato | 11 |
| Garlic | 12 | Vanilla | 9 |
| Lemon | 9 | Mustard | 10 |
| Wheat | 19 | | |

other foods that may be allergenic in nature. To reach a specific diagnosis, it is necessary to stress some peculiarities of food allergy.

First, we need to consider the *cyclic response*. If a patient is sensitive to a food which he eats regularly, he tends to become more sensitive to that food. If a food is omitted from his diet for a time, the patient may develop a tolerance for the food. When such a food is eaten after a prolonged abstinence, a reaction may not occur. However, if the food is again eaten frequently over a period of several days, an allergic reaction will probably reoccur.

Second, on the list is the *masked response*. When a food is eaten and causes a reaction, a second eating of the food while the reaction is occurring might diminish the reaction temporarily. However, after a few hours of relief, the symptoms will return. Cyclic and masked responses are possible and because of this attention should be focused on the foods a patient eats frequently, not the ones the patient rarely eats.

The patient must be free or nearly free of all symptoms before testing for allergies by food challenge will produce meaningful results. To accomplish this state of well being, two methods can be used. One method is to place the patient in a hospital in a controlled environment where the variables can be closely monitored. A second method is to place the patient on a diet consisting of foods the patient has never eaten or foods he infrequently eats. If a patient has never eaten a food, he cannot be allergic to it. If the patient seldom eats a food, there is a chance he is not allergic to it. The diet method advantage in cost to the patient is that it can be done at home. Still, diets vary with individual people and the areas where they live. A food the patient eats as often as once a week or every two weeks should be eliminated from participation on the elimination diet.

The following list of foods has been effective in eliminating symptoms:

## DIET FOR FOUR FULL DAYS ( 1 )

| | |
|---|---|
| Meat | Seafood (fish, shrimp, tuna salmon, etc.), lamb, quail, duck, rabbit, squirrel, wild game (deer, goat, etc.) |
| Vegetables | Sweet potato, broccoli, cauliflower, spinach, turnips,  beets, asparagus, okra, squash, greens, carrots |
| Fruits | Plums, pears, pineapple, grapes, bananas, nectarines, prunes, raisins, canned fruit (water packed) |

## DIET FOR FOUR FULL DAYS (2)

| | |
|---|---|
| Starches/Cereals | Rice, oatmeal, barley cereal, banana flakes |
| Bread | Kavli Norwegian Crispbread, (Rye, Red Box), rice wafers |
| Sweets | Artificial sweeteners or honey (no beet or cane) |
| Drinks | Del Monte or Dole pineapple juices (unsweetened), Welch's grape juice (unsweetened) |
| Salt | Sparingly |

Suggestion: eat a new food on an empty stomach daily or five times daily and check reactions. If you eat a new food on an empty stomach, you will react within two hours if you are allergic to that food. Things to watch for in your reactions: asthma, cough, post nasal drip, nasal congestion, sneezing, gas, indigestion, bloating, headache, hives, eczema, and so on.

Add a new food every three or more hours. If a reaction occurs after eating a food, take four tablespoons milk of magnesia for an adult (120 or more pounds), and take less in proportion for children. If the reaction does not clear, delay the next feeding until it does.

Kinds and amounts are listed below:

| | |
|---|---|
| Sugar | Diet sugar may be used |
| Wheat | Cream of Wheat |
| Chocolate | 2 tablespoons cocoa |
| Baker's Yeast | 1 teaspoon powdered, dissolved in 2 oz. of warm water |
| Peanut | 1 bag, salted |
| Corn | Grits |
| Mustard | 2 tablespoons |
| Vanilla | 1 teaspoon, extract |
| Cinnamon | 1 teaspoon |
| Lemon | 2 lemons |
| Shellfish | Shrimp, crab, oyster |
| Food color | Diet Grape Shasta |
| Caramel | Tab cola |
| Soybeans | 1 tablespoon, usually found in health store |

This diet is more liberal than the diet usually suggested, but it was found that patients are more likely to stick with it in this format and less likely to take liberties. If a patient is allergic to foods and follows this diet for four or five days, all. his allergy symptoms should clear up. If improvement does not occur, then the patient may be allergic to one of the foods allowed in the elimination diet, or the patient may not have followed the diet completely (some, as an example, refuse to give up coffee, tea, or some other item), or the patient may also be allergic to various inhalants which cause symptoms that mask any improvement resulting from the diet, or chemical gases often found in industrialized areas may be causing an allergic reaction which can mask improvement.

Once the symptoms have been controlled, challenge feeding of new foods (foods not on the elimination diet) can begin. This is a process that a patient can do at home by himself. A patient can best do this by staying home (perhaps on weekends) and testing four to six foods each day. However, a patient can continue his regular daily schedule and reduce testing to two or three foods a day.

The following example shows the challenge feeding test method at work. If breaking the diet starts at 9 a.m., the patient should drink 12 ounces of orange juice at this time. If the patient is allergic, he will react within two hours with usual symptoms. If the patient's usual complaints are nasal symptoms and bronchial asthma, he may develop nasal blockage with some discharge, or perhaps begin sneezing after drinking the orange juice. If the lung is sensitized, asthma symptoms will develop along with nasal symptoms.

After the symptoms are completely controlled and eliminated, a second food challenge can be done. The patient might try milk. If no reaction occurs within two hours, the patient is not allergic to milk! Patients are generally advised to wait an additional hour to allow the stomach to empty and to make sure no delayed reactions occur before the next test.

A reaction may last from hours to a day or two, so proper methods must be used to stop the attack. The patient must be free of symptoms before additional tests can be done.

If the patient does not improve on the diet given, any one or all four factors may be the failure cause. The patient should then be hospitalized in a controlled environment.

# 20

# *ENVIRONMENTAL CONTROL*

Environmental control for diagnosis and treatment of allergic conditions was initiated by Dr. Theron Randolph of Chicago and involves total control of the patient's food, air, water, and general surroundings. This procedure is used when a patient cannot be effectively evaluated in the doctor's office or patient's home.

Environmental factors, including inhalants such as house dust mites, pollens, molds, and animal dander, can aggravate and mask allergic reactions in sensitive patients when food is also a factor. Gases in the air around industrialized areas can mask the allergy under investigation. Frequently, a patient may be allergic to gases produced by synthetics such as polyester pillows, Dacron and nylon clothes, foam rubber pillows and mattresses. These environmental factors can obscure the allergy picture and must be eliminated in order to effectively evaluate foods related to allergies.

The best way to eliminate or control these factors is to place the patient on a therapeutic fast in a place where the air is free of particulate matter such as pollens, molds, dusts, and dander, and has been screened of hydrocarbons and other gases such as sulphur dioxide. In such a program, all synthetic materials are eliminated along with cosmetics, flowers, and odorous soaps. Creating such a controlled environment seems difficult, but it is manageable. Plain soaps and hard plastics, like those found in table tops or radios and televisions, are permitted. A mixture of salt and soda is a good toothpaste substitute. All cleaning fluids used in the patient's room must be free of odors. Plain, unscented soap and water suffice. All freshly printed material is eliminated, but old books, magazines, and papers are also permitted.

As stated earlier, I began my practice in Port Arthur, Texas, and St. Mary's Hospital in that city was the site for the controlled environment we needed to effectively isolate patient allergies. Port Arthur is heavily petrochemically industrialized and has a pre-dominance of sulphur dioxide in the air. Hydrocarbons are not a major factor in the air due to the environmental control efforts of the various industries in the area and stern monitoring by federal agencies. But the sulphur dioxide concentration remained high.

A word here about ventilation. The hospital ventilation at St. Mary's was nearly perfect. Special bags removed 98.5 per cent of the particulate matter, and down to 0.3 of a micron. A micron is 1/25,000 of an inch. This is smaller than a germ, and so the hospital was kept free of germs, dusts, molds, pollens, and other similar matter. After the air was filtered through the screening bags, it passed additionally through running water which absorbed most of the air gases.

But when a general system as just described is not available, an air purifier with two charcoal and two purafil filters can be used with a reasonable degree of confidence. The air purifier system also can have a high-fidelity filter which removes 95 per cent of particulate matter down to 0.3 micron. Electronic and other such machines will not remove **air** gases. The charcoal and purafil filters will. A window air conditioner is ideal because the same air is recirculated. A central air conditioning system is workable if the vent openings are partially closed to the point of minimal comfort.

The patient stays in this controlled room environment and is placed on a complete fast except for spring water. Spring water is used to eliminate chemicals such as sodium fluoride, chlorine, DDT, and other contaminants. Using a complete fast approach eliminates chance of error in uncovering a food allergy. When a limited diet fails to alleviate symptoms, environmental control and a fast can isolate the cause or causes of chronic illness.

If the patient is not too ill, the fast can be started the day before admittance to the hospital controlled environment. The patient takes the last meal between 4 p.m. and 5 p.m., and at bedtime takes four tablespoons of Milk of Magnesia to ensure intestinal elimination. Children take less of the magnesia in proportion to weight. A 150-pound adult takes a dose of four tablespoons, compared to a 75-pound child who takes two tablespoons. Only spring water is allowed after the patient's admittance. The fast continues until there is complete relief of symptoms.

Patients who are only allergic to inhalants and/or gases in the air will clear up in two to three days. Patients who are sensitive to foods will cease to have symptoms in three to five days. Patients allergic to chemicals such as pesticides in foods will clear up in six to nine days. Improvement in chemical allergy cases takes longer because the chemicals are stored in fatty body tissues. As the patient loses weight, chemicals are released from the fat. This release may cause an aggravation of symptoms in a patient who is allergic to them! Symptoms occurring during fasting can be controlled by medication.

After one or two days of fasting, acidosis develops which causes some degree of fatigue as well as a sense of well being or euphoria. After the third day of fasting, anorexia or loss of appetite is common.

A note on liquid intake. The patient is supplied with spring water and told to drink at least two to three quarts in 24 hours. Alkaline water is also supplied. This consists of two parts sodium bicarbonate and one part potassium bicarbonate. Each 8-ounce glass contains about one teaspoon of this mixture. This alkaline solution is used to stop attacks of allergic symptoms brought on by a food the patient proves to be allergic to and once challenge feeding or testing of foods begins. The alkaline solution causes an intestinal evacuation, ridding the intestines of any remnants of the particular food which caused the allergic attack. Also, it neutralizes the cellular acidity which results from an allergic attack and so stops the attack within 30 minutes to two hours, in most cases. After this period, another food can be used to challenge the patient. Children find this alkaline solution distasteful, so Milk of Magnesia can be given as a substitute (again, four tablespoons is an adult dose).

If nausea, with or without vomiting, excess hunger or fatigue occurs, even after the first day of fasting, the patient should be given a glucose solution intravenously. This controls all such symptoms, and the patient no longer feels anxiety or stress. This can be repeated daily or every other day should circumstances warrant. For children, this fasting technique works wonderfully well, but they should be given intravenous fluids daily or every other day during the fast before evidence of stress appears.

Glucose is safe to use under such circumstances as the material is corn sugar and almost completely nonallergenic. It will not cause reactions in patients allergic to corn.

The fast may be broken when the symptoms of allergy are nearly or completely relieved for 12 or more hours without the use of medication. To break the fast, start with foods that are eaten by the majority of people about once a week. Occasional changes in diet are necessary depending upon the food habits of individual patients. For the most part, the patient is challenged on 40 items consisting of foods, condiments, and food additives, such as color and caramel.

The foods and additives have been discussed in a previous chapter. Four days of fasting usually suffices for most patients. Frequently, small children clear up in two to three days. If symptoms have cleared in that period of time, the fast is broken. BUT DON'T USE FOODS EATEN THE DAY BEFORE THE FAST BEGAN. The foods used at the start of feeding should not have been eaten during the prior four days. Reactions are more marked if the food eaten has not been in the diet for four days. This phenomenon was first described by the famous researcher, Rinkle.

If a patient is allergic to a food which has been removed from the diet for at least four days, he will usually react to that food within two hours. An extra hour should be allowed for observation between tests in case of a delayed reaction.

Break the fast at 9 a.m. with 12 ounces of orange juice, a lesser amount suffices for a child. If a reaction occurs (nasal, bronchial, gastrointestinal, central nervous system, or skin symptoms), the patient must drink three glass of alkaline water at once. If the alkaline mixture is not tolerated, four tablespoons of Milk of Magnesia can be substituted. In most cases, the symptoms subside before the next scheduled feeding. If symptoms persist, all further feedings must be cancelled until complete relief is obtained. Attacks can last 48 hours in some cases and should be treated by medication. As testing progresses, if the patient gets hungry, feed foods previously tested and found to be nonallergic. If the patient is well before the noon feed is due, 15 ounces of milk (test item) is administered. If no reaction occurs by 3 p.m., broiled beef is ordered. Sea salt can be used at will. At 6 p.m., oatmeal is given, and at 9 p.m. two tablespoons of sugar can be served. Feedings are resumed at 6 a.m. the next morning and progress every three hours.

The majority of patients are able to average five feedings a day. If beef, chicken, or pork fail to cause trouble, the patient can eat them again, but with excess black pepper, red pepper, garlic, or with a raw or cooked onion, string beans, and so forth. This allows for the convenient testing of condiments. Food color is given in the form of a diet Grappette bottled drink which contains the three major food colors found in our food supply: blue #1, red #42, and yellow #5. Caramel is given in a diet cola bottled drink. Tab cola is best as it does not contain food color which some drinks contain. Cottonseed and safflower oil can be given in one ounce amounts by fast swallowing. An orange juice chaser can be used if such juice has been tested and tolerated.

The patient who clears of symptoms at home using the elimination diet discussed in the last chapter breaks the diet by food challenges as is done in the hospital. A patient may not be able to break his usual routine on the outside (not hospitalized), in which case, due to inconvenience or inopportunity, the patient can limit food challenges to once or twice a day throughout the week and increase the tests to several times a day on weekends.

When the symptoms of hospitalized patients do not clear until the sixth day of fasting or later, it means the patient is sensitive to chemical contaminants in foods. In order to avoid confusion regarding this issue, challenge feedings must be done with foods that have been organically grown and kept free from pesticide residues, preservatives, and other chemical contaminants. When the routine testing of organic foods is completed, the same foods must be retested using produce from the regular market. When the patient is allergic to pesticide residues and chemical contaminants of foods, symptoms return after the ingestion of foods from the market that had circumvented the organic testing program. At that point, a return to the organic diet is essential for recovery.

The patient also is tested for sensitivity to newsprint (newspapers), cosmetics, plastics, and rubber foam. The patient is instructed to smell each item thoroughly for five minutes or less if a reaction occurs. All testing stops with the first reaction and then restarted 30 minutes before a subsequent feeding. A reaction usually subsides within 15 to 20 minutes. Allergy to rubber foam, polyester pillows, or synthetic clothes usually requires contact from 30 to 60 minutes to be sure of a sensitivity.

Once the testing regime is successfully completed and the patient is discharged from the hospital, he is instructed to follow his diet carefully so that the clinical course can be evaluated. About 8 per cent of patients who resided in the area where my office was located developed symptoms due to airborne chemicals or gases, such as sulphur dioxide. When that occurred, the patient was isolated in his bedroom with a rented air purifier. He stayed in the room with doors and windows closed while following the diet established from the hospital testing. Within two to three days, relief of symptoms occurred if such symptoms were caused by an allergy to gases. When this was the case, the patient returned to normal living as long as the air purifier was used at least eight continuous hours at night. Since it usually took one to four days for a patient to accumulate a high enough concentration of gases in his system to produce symptoms, filtering the air at night usually sufficed to maintain remission.

If the patient returns home and develops symptoms the first night he is probably allergic to chemicals in his home. This can be checked by smelling each chemical, such as cleaning fluids, cosmetics and so on, for five minutes or less to determine what causes a reaction.

Some case studies are offered to clarify the point. Robert Muldowney, a 55-year-old mailman and having the same route in Austin for over 30 years, came to my office with chronic nasal allergy of long duration. Tests for inhalants were negative. An elimination diet also proved negative. Hospitalization for a therapeutic fast was ordered, and complete relief followed. Challenge feedings involved four foods. Upon discharge from the hospital, Robert developed symptoms the first night back home. This indicated that we needed to take a hard look at his household chemicals. The next day, Robert checked all items at home. By direct contact, he developed symptoms of headache and nasal congestion from perfumed candles as well as three household cleansers. Upon removal of these inhalants and four foods, Mr. Muldowney experienced complete and lasting relief.

Harvey Oldman had been retired for nearly 30 years when he came to see me in the mid '70's. He was in great shape for an 85-year-old, but he complained of significant asthma of two years' duration. Previous to that, he had experienced only mild respiratory allergy of negligible significance. It was assumed that the severe asthma was precipitated by the loss of his wife which was a great emotional blow. Tests for inhalants were negative. Hospitalization in St. Mary's showed that he was free of reaction from chemicals and other contaminants. On a therapeutic fast, he cleared in three days. He was also negative to food challenges. Within two days after returning home, Harvey's asthma returned. A diagnosis of sulfur dioxide allergy was made, and he was then isolated to his room for three days with an air purifier mediated by purafil and charcoal filters. He was completely well by the third day. By use of this special machine, he lived a good life for another five years until he died of unrelated causes. Such a machine must be kept up by replacing the charcoal and purafil filters every two to three months, OR WHEN NEEDED, depending upon the severity of atmospheric conditions about the patient's city.

Margaret Connally, a 70-year-old woman with bronchial asthma of many years, came to my clinic one day hardly able to breathe.

Previous therapy was of no avail. She proved negative to inhalants such as dust, molds, and so on. She was hospitalized in a clean environment, and her symptoms completely cleared in two days! All foods proved negative. Upon questioning her in depth, I found that she used pine oil in her home for general purposes. Pine oil was then ordered for test purposes by having her smell the oil in the container. Severe asthma attacks followed. Her relatives then thoroughly cleaned her home of all pine oil, its odor, and all pine oil bottles were removed. Mrs. Connally then returned home from St. Mary's, clinically cured of asthma.

Not too many years ago a 35-year-old female, Dusty Morgan, came to my office complaining of chronic headache of nearly five years Duration. A country singer by trade, headaches had been getting worse, and she had seen several prominent doctors in the San Antonio area. She stated that the headache usually became significant after bedtime, but, upon awaking in the morning, the headache was even worse. During the day, Dusty's discomfort was less. This signalled the concern that the problem somehow originated in the bedroom. She slept on synthetic pillows. During those years of my allergy practice, six cotton pillows were kept in the office at all times to loan out to patients suspected of an allergy to synthetics. She took two pillows to use that particular night. If good results followed, she could keep the pillows. Remember, all tests for inhalants proved negative. The following morning Dusty gave me a call and reported that for the first time in years she felt really wonderful, that she had a great night's sleep, free, of any headache. This was the quickest cure to date. Synthetic pillows were not an uncommon cause of trouble, but, still, not a 100 per cent etiological factor.

# 21

## *HYDROCARBONS AND OTHER GASES AS RELATED TO THE FIELD OF ALLERGY*

Patients with respiratory allergy, including nasal and bronchial allergy, may be allergic to gases found in the air in industrialized areas. Hydrocarbon and sulfur dioxide gases CAN CAUSE ill effects in some respiratory allergy patients.

Most people will react to relative large quantities of these gases simply because of their irritating effects. Some, however, are unusually susceptible and develop symptoms from minute quantities which do not bother the average person.

Patients who are allergic to inhalants and/or food often notice their symptoms get worse after exposure to the chemical environment. After controlling their symptoms by eliminating offending food and inhalants, these same patients may find that small amounts of air pollutants do not affect them. It is imperative to distinguish those patients who are specifically allergic to one or more gases from those only secondarily affected by such gases.

Testing patients for sensitivity to gases can be done by directly exposing the patient to a concentrated source of the gas. Under clinical control conditions (a study), 180 patients with perennial respiratory allergy were given provocative nasal tests with automobile exhaust fumes. Patients were placed in close proximity to such fumes for 60 seconds or less. If symptoms failed to occur within five minutes, the test was considered negative. Objective symptoms included cough, post nasal drip, nasal congestion, and wheezing. Subjective symptoms were headache, dizziness, weakness, and nausea. Of the 180 patients tested in this manner, 27 or 15 per cent reacted with objective symptoms. A concentrated automobile exhaust extract was made by bubbling exhaust fumes through extracting fluid. This extract was used successfully to test and treat patients found allergic to gases produced by automobiles. Most patients with identified allergies to automobile exhaust gases achieved an immunity to these gases after two to three months of injections.

While the automobile accounts for 80 per cent of the air pollution in Los Angeles County, California, the major air pollutant in southeast Texas with its petrochemical industries is sulphur dioxide. Patients with allergy to atmospheric gases cleared when isolated in an environmentally controlled room. Over a period of years, my office tested approximately 150 patients who were highly allergic to chemically polluted air. Twenty of these patients, about 13 per cent, were allergic only to sulphur dioxide. For these twenty patients, near or complete relief of symptoms was accomplished through use of a special air purifier in the patient's sleeping room. Most of the 150 patients were also allergic to substances such as food or inhalants in addition to the chemical air pollutants. In these cases, the use of an air purifier was definitely indicated.

To have the patient relocate to an area of clean air would not have always produced sufficient benefit to justify the inconvenience and expense. For those special patients, it is important to determine the food and inhalants that contribute to the overall allergic picture before addressing the problem of chemical air pollution. However, the tests for foods and inhalants cannot be carried out in the office while the patient remains at home because the patient's sensitivity to chemical air pollutants prevents him from clearing of symptoms no matter how appropriate the elimination diet. Such patients can only be evaluated by hospitalization in an area with clean air. Only in this way can food and other antigens causing the patient's allergic symptoms be accurately diagnosed and successfully treated.

Sulphur dioxide (SO2) is an allergy factor in about 8 per cent of all patients I have seen while located in the Port Arthur, Texas, area. To test for a SO2 allergy, the patient must be confined in an area free of this gas. If the patient shows marked improvement or even freedom of symptoms in a nonindustrial area and trouble reoccurs within two days upon returning home, you can easily diagnosis that SO2 is the culprit. A trial treatment using an air purifier mediated by purafil and charcoal filters can be utilized. Have the patient stay in a closed room and air condition only with a window unit for approximately three days. If there is a clearing of symptoms, such symptoms return if the air purifier is removed.

The method used in Port Arthur, Texas, was to admit the patient into St. Mary's where the air intake system within the hospital was so constructed that the air inside the building was virtually free of the SO2 gas. The patient was put on a therapeutic fast and, if cleared in four days, food challenges were made. If food was involved, the patient was discharged on a specialized diet. If trouble then surfaced upon immediate discharge, then you could pretty well bet that chemicals in the air within the home were the culprits. If trouble occurred within two days but not immediately upon arriving home, then SO2 was suspected. A further note here about the purifying system at St. Mary's. The air entering the hospital went through bags which captured all particles as stated previously, .3 microns or larger. Thus, pollens and molds were eliminated. Then the air went through water which absorbed gases. In this way, the air within the confines of the hospital was pure. All hospitals do not have such a wonderful, effective system, even to this day.

An interesting side, note. Chemical air pollution is not limited to the outdoors, as previously hinted. Indoor air pollution in the form of household gas has a definite role in the field of allergy and ecological illness. When gas is burned openly in pilot lights, gas ranges, or stoves, usually complete combustion results. Such combustion occurred because the gas flame was blue throughout. However, when the flame has some pink or red in it, some amount of incomplete combustion occurs with the resulting escape of hydrocarbons. Because household gas is odorless, ethylmercaptan is added to give a warning odor should gas escape. This product, like gas itself, is burned to yield carbon dioxide, water, and sulphur dioxide. However, most symptoms result from allergy to the hydrocarbons of the gas, itself.

Patients are checked for sensitivity to utility gas by having them smell escaping gas from an open gas vent in my medical office. In several patients, the gas precipitated asthma in as little as three seconds. Let's face it, no home utilizing gas as a heating source is totally free of gas leaks. This leak may be minor as far as the health of a nonsusceptible patient is concerned, but his minor leak will cause chronic or acute illness in a susceptible patient. In many instances, the gas company engineer can't locate and thus smell or otherwise find a very small leak. But this tiny problem can have a disastrous impact on the susceptible patient.

103

Another gas of prominence is chlorine. This gas, in the form of calcium chloride, is used as a disinfectant in our water supply, and not just in isolated areas but everywhere. The chlorine is in a concentration of abut two parts per million. In swimming pools, the concentration is approximately five parts per million. So, with this comparison, you get some idea how toxin chlorine in drinking water can be. Clorox bleach, which contains sodium hypochlorite, is a source of pure chlorine. A diagnosis is made by letting the patient smell Clorox for up to five minutes. If allergy to chlorine exists, a reaction occurs. The reaction may consist of congestion, post nasal drip, coughing, or wheezing. Further, a patient who is allergic to chlorine can safely drink water which has been brought to a boiling point to evaporate the chlorine. Water from the tap can also be dechlorinated by exposing a pitcher of this water to sunlight for a few hours. Injection therapy is most effective in immunizing patients allergic to chlorine, with significant improvements occurring within a few months. Such immunization allows patients to use any chlorinated water.

# 22

# THE RELATIONSHIP OF FOOD, DRUG, AND COSMETIC DYES TO RESPIRATORY ALLERGY

Food coloring is used in many packaged, canned and bottled foods primarily for psychological effect to make the product look more appealing, therefore, effecting greater sales. Everyone ingests some quantity of food dyes which may have some serious physical consequences. NO QUESTION WHATSOEVER exists that these artificial colors play a role in the field of allergy.

Interest in this field occurred some years ago when one of my patients was hospitalized for a therapeutic fast and tests and reacted to a diet soft drink with symptoms of nasal allergy and asthma. The patient's sneezing, nasal congestion and wheezing occurred within 15 minutes of drinking a bottled diet grape drink. Although the beverage contained a conglomeration of preservatives, I assumed the dyes present were the allergens responsible for the allergic reaction.

Further investigation showed soft drinks contain the following food, drug, and cosmetic colors: *orange,* yellow #6, red #40; *cherry,* red #40; *raspberry,* red #40, blue *#1; grape,* red #40, blue #1, yellow *#5; strawberry,* red #40, yellow #6; lime, yellow #5, blue #1; *lemon,* yellow *#5; cola,* caramel color; and *Dr. Pepper,* caramel color. Bakery products make extensive use of colors in dough products, cookies, sandwich fillings, icings, and coatings. The high moisture content of doughs and batters makes the use of colors relatively easy. Caramel or carbon black is added to dark chocolate pieces along with combinations of certified (federally approved) colors.

Ice cream cones at one time were colored with water-soluble annato seed. However, certified colors are now used because they are more cost effective and offer a greater variety of colors. Generally, ice cream cones contain yellow #5 and #6. Nearly all ice creams and sherbets contain artificial color. Chocolate ice cream is often the exception. Annato is sometimes used in vanilla ice cream, but certified colors are increasingly popular.

Cheese is an insufficient staple for use in producing certified colors. Annato and B-carotene are the colorants of choice. Likewise, margarine and butter are chiefly colored with B-carotene and oil-soluble annato. It is hard to imagine candies, especially hard candy, without color. Red #40 is one of the most common colors used. The dry-mix products, such as gelatin desserts and puddings, often include red #40 and blue # 1. Medicines, themselves, contain a wide variety of artificial colors.

Caramel cannot be overlooked as a food color. This substance is an amorphous dark brown material resulting from the controlled heat treatment of food-grade carbohydrates: dextrose or glucose made from corn; invert sugar or sucrose made from cane or beets, lactose or milk sugar; malt syrup derived from barley; and molasses derived from all sugar. The caramel used in colas, root beer, most bakery foods, rye bread, and gravies is derived from corn. Icings of cakes use caramels made from cane sugar.

To confirm my assumption about the role of artificial colors in food allergy, I set about developing a mixture of dyes for provocative tests. My local supermarket in Port Arthur had available food, drug, and cosmetic dyes of yellow #5, red #40, and blue #1. With a concentrated mixture of these colors, I began to do routine testing. My test mixture addressed the most commonly used colors except yellow #6 and, initially, I used the sublingual technique, placing four drops under a patient's tongue, as the provocative testing method. After many trials, it was found that the sublingual test was about 30 per cent accurate. Direct feeding tests result in a much more accurate diagnosis and are now widely used.

Contrary to what you might want to think, studies show that allergy to food colors is quite common. In 500 consecutive patients under therapy for food, with or without inhalants, 15 per cent were allergic to food colors. Injection therapy produced immunity in most cases to food and food color allergy.

During my practice at Port Arthur, I had three asthmatic patients whose entire symptomology was caused by allergy to food color. It happens. These patients all had negative sublingual tests, but they reacted positively to challenge feedings of diet grape drink. All three cases responded to perfection with injection therapy. The patients, ages 57, 62, and 80, responded within three to five months of therapy as shown by negative reactions when challenged with 12 ounces of diet grape drinks. Before therapy, such challenges resulted in asthma attacks within 20 to 40 minutes.

At the 1974 allergy section meeting of the American Medical Association, Dr. Benjamin Feingold stressed the role played by food dyes and other chemical food additives in central nervous system allergy and its responsibility for the slow-learning syndrome in children.

Dr. Feingold, creator of the Feingold Diet, said that 85 per cent of the slow-learning children participating in the study had symptoms of nasal allergy, bronchial allergy, or both. He did not discuss the role food dyes play in cases of respiratory allergy.

From my experience of more than 50 years in the field of allergy, it is my opinion that dyes are usually not the sole cause of allergic reactions. The probability is quite high that the symptoms in Feingold's cases resulted from multiple food allergies. If these children had been checked by therapeutic fasting and challenge feedings, they would have shown respiratory system symptoms as well as central nervous system complications due to multiple food sensitivities.

# 23

# *ALLERGY AND EMOTIONS*

Depression, chronic fatigue, headaches, hyperactivity and hypoactivity are common emotional complaints within the general population of any society, especially today's hustle and bustle in the western world where you don't know from one day to the next if you'll still have a job the following week or whether the dollar on the world market will collapse by day's end. For years, these symptoms of the central nervous system have been released to the field of psychiatric medicine for treatment, while the field of allergy was limited to treating asthma, hay fever, and nasal problems. Today, however, it is known that the allergic syndrome may involve any area of the human system, including emotional complaints.

Psychologists and psychiatrists have done some spectacular work dealing with human emotions. But too often the use of drugs and/or long periods of therapeutic investigation have failed to alleviate many so-called emotional problems.

These patients are frequently misdiagnosed because the symptoms accompany organic diseases. Clear the organic maladies and the emotional symptoms may disappear. But a large number of people never get relief from their emotional symptoms because their symptoms are unrelated to organic disease! These people may lead productive lives, but they lack a great deal of luster.

These patients are truly the "Forgotten People," but they don't have to be. In every age group, these patients are curable if properly evaluated along allergic lines. In comparison to the time and expense involved with a psychological evaluation and treatment, an allergic investigation can be done quickly, without extensive or expensive tests, and without harm. For a patient with emotional symptoms, an allergic investigation should be among the first options explored rather than among the last. If the patient is free of allergic involvement, the analysis to arrive at that is harmless, quick, and inexpensive.

Depression, fatigue, hyper- and hypoactivity may be associated with asthma or nasal allergy, and these symptoms may be truly emotional based upon the associated physical aggravation of the bronchial and nasal airways. Clearing up the asthma may lead to mental relief, but far too frequently other specific allergens are responsible for the so-called mental symptoms. Also, these mental symptoms may be present without related physical problems of allergic origin.

The case of 31-year-old Sonja Smith comes to mind, a woman who had chronic headaches, fatigue, depression, aching teeth, and some gastrointestinal symptoms. When she came to my office in the late '70's, she had run the gambit of attempting to have her problem solved. There were no obvious allergy symptoms. Despite medical investigations, she did not get relief of her symptoms.

By chance, she read a book on allergy by Dr. Marshall Mandell of Norwalk, Connecticut, who had stressed the role allergy played in patients with emotional symptoms. She contacted two allergists who discouraged use of this approach. Since my name appeared in

Mandell's book, she telephoned me. Even though I was in a distant city from Sonja, I encouraged her in this allergic approach and suggested food allergy tests that she could do herself at home. It was suggested she follow a diet of spring water and a few foods that she seldom or never ate. She was to follow the diet for four days to allow time to eliminate all previously consumed foods from her system that might cause her symptoms.

On the fifth day, the woman called and happily reported that she was free of all her complaints! She was then directed to add foods back into her diet at the rate of one every three to four hours until symptoms appeared. Once symptoms appeared, she was to eliminate that food from her diet and continue testing.

Two weeks later, Sonja called with the following report:

| | | |
|---|---|---|
| 1) | Corn | = depression |
| 2) | Irish Potato | = fatigue |
| 3) | Orange (citruses) | = toothaches |
| 4) | Apple | = intestinal symptoms |
| 5) | Lettuce | = headache |
| 6) | Wheat | = swelling in throat |
| 7) | Rice | = headache |
| 8) | Shrimp | = headache |

The patient eliminated the foods involved from her diet, and she was advised that if she was still well in one week to retest the offending food for accuracy. A month later she reported that she tried each food three times, and all three times she experienced the same adverse reactions! This is an example of long-distance medicine as well as evidence of a clinical cure!

John Haney, a 30-year-old civil servant at the Johnson Space Center in Houston, had a different set of problems. He had been treated ten years previously for chronic nasal allergy associated with headache, depression, fatigue, nasal congestion, and neck-muscle pain. He was hospitalized for a therapeutic fast. He cleared of all symptoms in four days. When tested for food association, he reacted to five of them. He was then tested at my clinic after release from the hospital for inhalant factors. Provocative nasal tests produced positive reactions to house dust mites and several molds. Specific therapy for the mites and molds along with a proper diet produced perfect results. Mr. Haney took treatments for five years with perfect relief and continued free of symptoms for five more years without treatment. THEN, THE SAME SYMPTOMS RETURNED. After dealing with the problem for two months on his own, Mr. Haney called. By phone, he was placed on a limited diet for five days. At the end of the fifth day, he reported complete relief. He then started testing food, and again five foods were involved: corn, headaches; coffee, neck muscle ache; chocolate, fatigue and depression; sugar, nasal congestion; and lettuce, depression. He was retested for the inhalants that had previously caused symptoms. Provocative ophthalmic tests were still positive confirming allergies to mites and molds, but provocative nasal tests were negative, indicating the man was still successfully immunized against these inhalant factors. A diet change again resulted in a clinical cure from emotional symptoms.

A case such as John's is not unusual. People with undiagnosed ailments may live useful lives, but all too often not productive ones. The point is crucial: ENOUGH SUCCESSES HAVE BEEN LOGGED TO INITIATE A NEW TREND IN ALLERGY INVESTIGATION.

# 24

## ALLERGY AND THE CENTRAL NERVOUS SYSTEM

The Great Imitator's role: ALLERGY CAN PRODUCE SYMPTOMS IN ANY ORGAN OF THE BODY, INCLUDING THE CENTRAL NERVOUS SYSTEM (CNS). Allergy of the CNS causes edema or swelling of the brain which reduces the brain's blood supply and limits its ability to function normally.

The researcher Philpott wrote that this swelling typically leads to symptoms of either over- or under-response. That is, there may be hyperkinesis or hypokinesis, psychomotor excitement or retardation, mania or depression, hyperalertness or hypoalertness, insomnia or drowsiness, headache, or lightheadedness.

Many patients with CNS allergy also have some evidence of respiratory allergy. Therefore, it is important to perform a complete allergy investigation on any patient who has any CNS symptoms along with nasal or bronchial allergy symptoms. If a patient with cerebral symptoms has any evidence of respiratory allergy, regardless of its significance, this should be considered as having CNS allergy unless some other cause for the symptoms is found.

The effects of CNS allergy can be dramatic. Allergic reactions, in general, may interfere with the maturation of tissues. In chronic CNS allergy, the allergy interferes with the maturation of the CNS. A delay in CNS maturation is one source of dyslexia which can range from minor to major learning disabilities. Learning is interrupted, leading the child to feelings of frustration, anger, anxiety, and failure.

CNS ALLERGY IS NOT A NEW CONCEPT. In 1898, the researcher Baker described fatigue in school children as being food-related. Rowe further showed a definite relation between food allergy and CNS function. Randolph, Speer, and Mandell have discussed the relationship of food and chemicals to CNS allergy.

Bottom line: THE MOST COMMON CAUSE OF CNS ALLERGY IS FOOD. Chemicals and food additives also may play a significant role and must be considered in every case. My tests indicate that while patients may be sensitive to inhalants, such items play a minor role in CNS allergy symptoms. However, inhalants should be investigated along with food, chemicals, and additives. Provocative tests have shown that each allergen may produce symptoms in a different organ. Inhalants may produce respiratory symptoms, chemicals and additives may cause CNS symptoms and food may produce respiratory and CNS symptoms. It is clear that any combination of symptoms may exist.

Determining the specific allergen that produces the symptoms is of utmost importance in diagnosing CNS allergy AND THE ONLY WAY TO OBTAIN THAT SPECIFICITY IS BY USING THE PROVOCATIVE TESTING METHOD. To get an exact diagnosis, the patient should be hospitalized in a controlled atmosphere for therapeutic fasting. If a patient fasts for four to five days in a controlled environment and his CNS symptoms do not clear, then, the CNS symptoms probably are not due to allergy. If the fast clears up the respiratory symptoms, then, those allergens can be identified and treated. If hospitalization is impractical, the use of a limited diet for four or five days can well be the answer. If the fast relieves the symptoms, then challenge feeding begins. With hospitalized patients and those using limited diets at home, tests producing subjective symptoms must be repeated without the patient's knowledge to get accurate results.

Once the allergens are identified, treatment for CNS allergy can produce positive results. One such case involved Marty Akins, a three-year-old, hyperactive child in New Orleans who had been treated by a psychiatrist and an allergist for a year without improvement. It was at that point that Marty first came to see me. Provocative tests for inhalants proved negative. He was hospitalized and put on a therapeutic fast. His symptoms cleared in three and a half days! Challenge feeding produced nasal, bronchial, and CNS symptoms. His symptoms were caused by peanuts, fish, and food coloring. He was placed on a diet eliminating these items and was cured.

Another patient, Johnny Hightower of Tulsa, Oklahoma, age six, had only CNS symptoms of hyperactivity and slow learning, classic and not unusual. He was placed on a limited diet for four days at home, and his mother called my office on the afternoon of the fourth day, ecstatic over his overall improvement, especially his attention span. He only reacted violently to peanuts by oral challenge. The test for peanuts was repeated, and the adverse reaction again occurred. Johnny is now on a peanut-free diet and no longer takes medication for hyperactivity. Note: his previous diet included peanut butter on his school sandwiches which he ate every day.

# 25

# *GASTROINTESTINAL ALLERGY*

Gastrointestinal symptoms are a common complaint of patients seeking medical help, and this possible link to allergy is very often overlooked. These patients may have symptoms of excessive gas, flatulence, distention, vague abdominal discomfort, mild to severe cramping, diarrhea, constipation, alternate diarrhea and constipation, indigestion, vomiting, rectal itching and bleeding.

Sometimes gallstones, peptic and gastric ulcers may be responsible for such symptoms. HOWEVER, A PATIENT COMPLAINING OF SOME OR ALL OF THESE SYMPTOMS MAY HAVE NO ORGANIC DISEASE OF THE GALL BLADDER OR GASTROINTESTINAL TRACT! Spastic colitis is the most common diagnosis when no organic disease if found, and the patient is generally treated with a bland diet, antispasmodic medicines and tranquilizers which may provide some relief. Problems related to gallstones can be solved by removing the gall bladder. Ulcers can be treated with diet and medications. Such actions, though, may result in only partial relief of symptoms.

Most patients in this category are labelled neurotic, but the majority of patients with persistent symptoms have gastrointestinal allergy! They may suffer for years before having the good fortune of getting a complete allergic investigation, if at all!

Some degree of respiratory allergy usually surfaces in patients with gastrointestinal allergy. These patients have headaches, nasal congestion, post nasal drip, hacking cough, frequent sore throats, frequent upper respiratory flare-ups, so-called bronchial-pneumonia attacks, and even asthma. The researcher Siegal studied the relationship of gastrointestinal ulcers to allergy and found that 53 out of 54 patients with X-ray evidence of ulcers had respiratory allergy symptoms! Certainly, any patient with any degree of so-called "sinus" or respiratory allergy who reports gastrointestinal symptoms should have a thorough allergic investigation. Similarly, any patient with gastrointestinal symptoms not related to organic disease should undergo an allergic investigation.

Inhalants, such as house dust mites, pollens, molds, and animal danders may have some role in the "sinus" symptoms, but food is generally the cause of the nasal and gastrointestinal symptoms. However, the patient histories and skin tests used by traditional allergists are not accurate enough to result in a clinical cure or even near cure. Provocative allergy testing can, however, lead to such cures.

A patient in this category should be hospitalized for evaluation. Ulcers or gallstones, if found, should not be considered the final answer because a related gastrointestinal allergy is probably involved. Regardless of whether gallstones or ulcers are involved, the patient should be placed in a controlled environment and started on a therapeutic fast. Respiratory and gastrointestinal symptoms subside for most patients after a three- to five-day fast. Food challenges then can be made to determine the food involved. Later, provocative nasal and skin tests for inhalants can be done.

By way of illustration, I remember very well four cases in the late '70's on this issue, and they are cited here for the purpose of acquainting the reader with what can happen. These patients were hospitalized for therapeutic fasts and had upper respiratory and gastrointestinal symptoms with X-ray evidence of peptic ulcers that refused to heal. After eliminating the offending food from their diets, all symptoms were either completely cleared or under acceptable control. The fourth patient, 67-year-old Philip Martin, a retired real estate broker in the Houston area, came to me as a bona fide textbook example, still having multiple intestinal symptoms despite having had his stomach removed four years earlier! I hospitalized Mr. Martin immediately, as he suffered from chronic edema and intermittent lower abdominal distention with a lack of urinary control due to the resulting pressure. A series of gastrointestinal tests proved negative, but a routine gall bladder X-ray showed multiple stones. An allergic investigation implicated 12 different foods. Mr. Martin got complete relief of symptoms once these foods were eliminated from his diet! The large number of stones later indicated removal of his gall bladder.

Another cause of gastrointestinal symptoms is digestive intolerance of a particular food such as milk. Sensitivity to milk varies somewhat between different ethnic groups, but, generally, between ten to forty per cent of the population may be intolerant to lactose (milk sugar) in milk! That may be a blow to the dairy industry, but, oh well... As a result, milk may cause varying degrees of diarrhea, gas, bloating, and discomfort. These people can tolerate buttermilk, yogurt, and hard cheese because the lactose has been converted to lactic acid! A two-hour lactose tolerance test can be used to determine if a patient has a digestive intolerance to milk. The test is similar to the glucose tolerance test used for obtaining a blood sugar curve for diagnosing diabetes or hypoglycemia. It is possible for a person to be intolerant and allergic to milk at the same time. If

118

an individual reacts to buttermilk and yogurt as well as milk, then, the patient is allergic to milk and intolerant to lactose!

It is a tragedy that many patient with "sinus" and gastrointestinal symptoms suffer for years because doctors do recognize allergy as the probable cause of the symptom. Again, many allergists fail to find an answer to such problems because they rely on skin tests for diagnosis!

As a result of inadequate diagnosis, patients all too often go from doctor to doctor trying multiple nostrums for relief These patients are usually diagnosed as spastic colitis, neurosis, just plain "nuts." A certain number wind up in the psychiatric department of some institution because depression and fatigue frequently are also associated with gastrointestinal symptoms. These truly are "The Forgotten People," but they do not have to bear the cross alone. HOPE is more than just a cheap word and is very attainable with proper allergy evaluation.

# 26

# *ARTHRITIS AND ALLERGY*

Allergy can account for many illnesses, and arthritis is no exception, including rheumatoid and osteoarthritis and general types of joint pain. The relationship between allergy and arthritis was given a most complete discussion by Dr. Marshall Mandell of Norwalk, Connecticut, in his 1984 book, *Lifetime Arthritis Relief System*.

An interesting note: THE ARTHRITIS FOUNDATION REPRESENTATIVES DENY ANY CONNECTION BETWEEN FOOD ALLERGY AND ARTHRITIS! The foundation has even refused to spend ANY of the millions of dollars allocated for arthritis research on controlled hospital studies involving allergy investigations!

The fact remains that many people suffer with arthritis and spend a fortune for treatment that produces little or no relief! All such patients deserve an allergic investigation which takes at the most ten to fourteen days. If a patient does not benefit, he loses only a few days of his life. If he gets relief, he has gained a new lease on life!

Allergic arthritis is almost completely due to food, chemicals in food, and/or food additives. Just as in investigating respiratory, gastrointestinal, or CNS allergy, the arthritis patient should be hospitalized for a therapeutic fast. Because of the nature of the ailment, the fast may take a day or two longer for symptoms to clear. If hospitalization is impossible, a limited diet also can produce results, though not as striking. After fasting for five to seven days, challenge feedings can begin to determine the food involved.

It has been my experience that allergic arthritis is frequently associated with nasal, bronchial, gastrointestinal, and CNS allergies. These conditions may be minor or major in nature. A thorough allergic investigation can lead to a cure or near cure of all symptoms, including allergic arthritis associated with other body systems.

The following are three arthritic case studies dealing with just such events. Molly Thoms of Durant, Oklahoma, a 53-year-old housewife, came to me in October of 1981 with a complaint of arthritis and sought advice concerning her problem. I had last seen her in the summer of 1979 when she had completed a successful specific allergy therapy for headaches and nasal allergy. She said she had endured painful swollen joints for two years which had progressed to the point of near incapacitation. The doctor she had been seeing for this malady from the summer of 1979 to when she came back to see me made a diagnosis of rheumatoid arthritis based upon clinical examination and blood tests. She had only taken aspirin for relief which only had helped a little. I asked Molly why she had not spoken about the problem to me two years before, when it had all started. She said SHE KNEW IT WAS NOT DUE TO AN ALLERGY and she did not want to bother me with her troubles as I was an allergy specialist. Molly was immediately placed on a diet of food NEVER OR INFREQUENTLY eaten. After five days of this diet, Molly's pain was almost completely relieved. Challenge feedings were ordered. One food, tomato, had caused generalized joint pains within an hour after ingestion! She waited a few days after the symptoms disappeared and then drank 15 ounces of tomato juice for a second trial. The symptoms dramatically reappeared! She was then placed on specific allergic therapy for tomato, and the food was completely eliminated from her diet. Now, over ten years later, Molly is still completely free of arthritis, and she can even tolerate tomatoes in small, reasonable amounts (such as a minute topping on a salad). If Molly eats three tomatoes a day for three or four days, moderate symptoms reoccur. Otherwise, Molly is clinically cured.

Another woman, Mitzi Downs, a 42-year-old secretary in Houston, was evaluated for chronic nasal and bronchial allergy AND ARTHRITIS. The arthritis involved the spine, arms, legs, and hands which had been troubling her for several years. She had been treated with various drugs with a diagnosis of degenerative and rheumatoid arthritis. No matter what she did, or what doctor prescribed what, relief was negligible. Mitzi was hospitalized for a therapeutic fast. After four days, all symptoms were relieved. Challenge feedings indicated that nasal and bronchial symptoms were brought on by beef, black pepper, orange, sugar, string beans, tea, garlic, vanilla, lemon, fish, shellfish, and cottonseed oil. Arthritic symptoms were produced by cinnamon, milk and pork. These three foods were frequently eaten in her everyday regular diet. A month later, after eliminating these foods from her diet, Mitzi was still free of arthritic symptoms. Granted, Mitzi proved allergic to a vast number of foods, much more so than most but elimination of these culprits from her eating patterns was her saving grace. Many other wonderful choices of food can be had as long as you know WHAT TO STAY AWAY FROM IN YOUR OWN PERSONAL SITUATION.

Dottie Morgan, a 74-year-old retired nurse of over 50 years in the Little Rock, Arkansas, area, had similar yet different problems. Dottie had a history of chronic nasal symptoms, including sneezing, nasal congestion, post nasal drip, CNS symptoms of moderately frequent frontal headaches, gastrointestinal problems of gas and bloating, and, you guessed it, ARTHRITIS. Her arthritic condition included the hands, wrists, elbows, and shoulders, which appeared with pain, increased heat, some swelling, and marked limitation of motion. She could close her fingers but could not make a fist. She could touch her face but could not reach behind her neck. Dottie had previously been diagnosed as having progressive rheumatoid arthritis which had begun ten years earlier. Dottie also had four years of gold therapy and was receiving injections every two weeks when she first came to see me in early 1981. She had been taking 12 to 16 tablets of Ecotrin (coated aspirin) daily, and the gold injections produced only slight improvement so she discontinued them. I hospitalized Dottie in March of that year for a therapeutic fast. After four days of fasting, there was almost complete relief from arthritic pain! The swelling left, and motion was restored without the use of pain medication. The improvement was remarkable because she would now make a fist then point her finger at me when making a conversational point. The nasal, CNS, and gastrointestinal symptoms had been completely relieved. Challenge feedings (culprit foods) reproduced all of her symptoms involving decreased use of the various bodily systems. She reacted to orange, sugar, pork, lemon, and tomato. She was happily discharged on a diet without medication, clinically cured! Six weeks later, Dottie's joint movement was still improving, and -she only had transient pain, able to be controlled with two to four tablets of Ecotrin taken only on occasional days.

Other case studies are available, but the fact remains that many chronic diseases are of AN ALLERGIC NATURE. If handled properly, a substantial number of these patients can get relief within ten to fourteen days with proper allergy therapy. If an allergy evaluation fails to produce results, the patient has only lost two weeks of time with no potentially dangerous medications having been used. This is a small price to pay, considering potential benefits.

What you have just read is, perhaps, the most controversial section of this book. Still, "sacred cows" aside, why should innocent patients seeking professional help at great expense to ease their pain be needlessly subjected to time-worn methods of so-called "doctoring" that do not have a chance in hell of ever succeeding? In Molly Thoms' case, she was told by a prominent physician to "take an aspirin and call me in the morning"! The choice is yours. Wake up and think.

We bring a lot of our own ills upon ourselves, and a lot of allergies come about as negative reactions to ingested food. I am ready and willing to defend every word in this chapter. Referring to those who maintain there is no connection between allergy and arthritis, are they ready and willing to defend erroneous positions they have held for years?

Not to beat a dead horse or impose any lifestyle on any person for any reason other than from a medical point of view, have you ever wondered why Seventh-day Adventists, health conscious members of the Jewish faith, and Mormons are much healthier individuals than the general populace? It is no secret. Watching what you eat and why is critical to healthful living and longevity. It is that simple. But when a person suffers through no fault of his own, such as from an unknown food allergy, it is up to doctors and the field of medicine at large to provide the most accurate and effective service to mankind, not hide behind shields of inconsequence.

You decide. It is your body.

# 27

# *FUNGAL INFECTIONS AND ID REACTIONS*

The body normally contains fungi that are nondisease producing (saprophytic). However, these fungi can become disease producing (pathogenic) under certain circumstances, causing fungal infections of the ear (external auditory canal), vaginal tract, nail beds, gastrointestinal tract, and skin.

Severe, debilitating disease such as uncontrolled diabetes, leukemia, or carcinoma can convert nondisease producing fungi to pathogens. Excessive use of antibiotics, steroids, and hormones can produce similar results.

More than one fungus may be involved, but monilia, albicans, or candida is the fungus or mold most commonly involved. Monilia albicans is so prevalent in our environment that it is not unusual to find this organism on the skin, in sputum, or in the vagina where it lives as a harmless saprophyte. Finding small numbers of such fungi at various times is of no importance and, under such circumstances, such fungi are not generally associated with infections. If cultures consistently produce rich growths of monilia, then, the fungus is acting as a true pathogen. In such cases, local therapy with antifungicides can produce excellent results when the medication can come into direct contact with the fungi involved such as in infections of the ear canal, gastrointestinal tract, skin, or vaginal tract. Athletes foot, for example, which is a fungal infection, can be treated effectively with medication. However, recurrences are frequent when the fungal infection penetrates into the deeper layers of the involved tissue where localized therapy cannot reach. This is especially likely in fungal infections of the nail bed or vagina.

Systemic fungicides can reach these deeper tissue layers and may be the complete answer. Immunologic therapy stimulates the body to produce blocking antibodies to attack the fungal infections. Ibis is like injections of diphtheria or tetanus vaccines which stimulate the formation of antibodies that destroy invading diptheria and tetanus germs.

In the past, fungi were not recognized as causing infections because routine cultures did not reveal possible fungal involvement. Therefore, if one suspects a fungus is involved in an infection, specific methods of investigation must be used. Doctors should use culture media that grows fungi without growing bacteria. Nickerson's Media can be used which grows monilia albicans at room temperature within 24 to 48 hours. This media grows other fungi in five to ten days.

A fungal infection in any of the body's systems may not only cause local symptoms but may act as a focus distributing toxins that cause allergic reactions known as dermatophytid or ID reactions. These reactions may appear in various forms ranging from a bumpy, itching skin rash to a severe, oozing eczema. Generally, ID reactions are defined as pustular or vesicular eruptions of the hands resulting from a focal fungal infection of the feet. In short, athlete's foot infection produces toxins in the body that cause the hands to break out with a rash or lesions. The solution is relatively simple: treat the athlete's foot and the rash on the hands will go away. The focal infection (athlete's foot, per the example) can be successfully treated by local or oral therapy. Griseofulvin, Mycostatin, Gentian Violet, Lotrimin, and Nizoral are successful oral and local medications that treat individual or groups of fungi.

Until now, I have discussed classic symptoms and reactions, but not all fungal infections and ID reactions are obvious. ID reactions concern focal or localized fungal infections that have invaded deeper cell layers such as the nasopharynx and the bronchial tree, and cannot be reached by local therapy. Problems in these areas also are less likely to be diagnosed as fungal in nature. ID reactions may appear without the skin blisters and rashes. ID reactions may resemble typical skin eruptions, fixed red spots or swollen, itchy patches on any area such as the neck, sacrum, face, or around the anus.

When local fungal infections cannot be reached by local therapy, oral therapy with medication designed for the fungus involved can be quite effective. Such distant lesions also can be treated successfully with immunological methods consistent with allergy therapy. Once the specific fungus causing the allergic ID reaction is identified, it can be treated like any other allergy. The specific allergen is injected deep under the skin to form antibodies which will attack invaders similar to those the injections contain.

In a series of 35 cases of focal monilia infections, there were five ID reactions involving anal dermatitis, sacral eczema (involving the skin at the end of the spine), eczema completely encircling the neck, and two cases of papular dermatitis of the face and neck. Scrapings of these lesions failed to grow fungi. Treatment with steroids gave excellent remissions with a week to ten days, but the lesions returned once the steroids were discontinued.

These five patients had focal monilial infections that I personally verified with three consecutive cultures taken several days apart. Each culture produced abundant monilia growths. The infections were in the external auditory canal, the vaginal tract, nasopharynx, and the dorsal area of one foot. The individual's fungal infections were treated with immunological therapy and the ID reactions disappeared two weeks after the fungal infections were controlled by injections.

The most common infection caused by monilia albicans occurs in the vaginal tract. Although oral medications cure the majority of such infections, a significant number recur. Immunological therapy can be the final answer to these recurrent types of infection. The normal flora of germs in the vagina may include many types of organisms including some pathogenic ones and, not infrequently, fungi of various sorts. However, my experience has shown that dealing with vaginal smears from noninfectious vaginas usually results in such organisms being generally absent or few in number with the exception of Doderlein's Bacilli. This is a normal vaginal bacilli found especially before menstruation. A culture is the only way to determine the normal, microscopic occupants of the vagina.

While the diagnosis of vaginitis is made easily enough by a simple inspection of the area, it is important to eliminate other causes of the problem before labeling it nonspecific vaginitis. In the adult, this means eliminating (as possible causes) trichomas and fungal infections which produce a clinical picture similar to nonspecific vaginitis.

Monilial or candida infection of the vagina is characterized by a discharge which varies between thin and watery to thick and purulent. Pruritus may be intense, and local irritation and marked reddening of the entire vaginal or vulva-vaginal membrane usually occurs. In addition, there may be white patches on the vagina, vulva, or both when the vulva is extensively involved.

While the picture described in the paragraphs above should suggest a mycotic etiology, a microscopic examination of the organisms present should be made to confirm the diagnosis. A culture of vaginal secretions should also be done. Frequent recurrences of this fungal infection should be treated by immunological methods.

Bottom line: IN TESTING A FEMALE PATIENT FOR ANY ALLERGY, THE ALLERGIST SHOULD QUESTION THE PATIENT ABOUT ANY RECURRING VAGINITIS. If there is evidence of a monilia infection and a history of recurrences, the allergist should add this to general therapy procedures.

Other fungal infections such as chronic external otitis media and of the nail beds should be searched for and, if present, included in therapy for allergies. If cultures cannot be made, such as in nail bed inflammatory conditions, the allergist should use a mixture of fungal antigens in therapy, such as a mixture of trichophyton, odiomyces, and epidermophyton. The trade name for these three fungi is TOE.

Let's get into two real cases that I dealt with in the early '80's to see how it works. Robert Hillman, a 40-year-old car salesman from Austin, Texas, came to see me with a ring of eczema around his neck of six months duration. Local therapy failed to provide relief. Evidence of nasal congestion and post nasal drip was present. Scrapings of eczema were free of bacteria and fungi. Nasal smears proved negative for allergy, but culture samples showed excessive growth of fungi, namely monilia albicans. Diagnosis centered on ID reactions, the focus of which was in the nasal passages. Treatment indicated an allergy basis with a vaccine of monilia albicans. Complete cure occurred within three months.

Mary Travers, a 30-year-old school teacher from Lubbock, Texas, had severe eczema of the sacral area (end of spine). Cultures proved negative for fungi. Chronic monilial vaginitis was found. The vaginal area was treated locally with a resultant cure of vaginitis followed by the disappearance of ID reactions on the sacrum. However, within two months the ID reactions recurred. Immunological (allergy) therapy was initiated and within three months both the eczema and vaginitis was cured. This therapy continued for one year, and Mary was clinically cured.

# 28

## *HIVES OR URTICARIAL DERMATOSIS*

Hives or urticaria and angioedema or general swelling of the skin are similar in origin and pathology and may be related to allergy. The hives and swelling, though, differ in location of the lesions.

Generally, hives are reddish or pinkish bumps on the skin that itch and burn. They may vary from minute lesions to large welts. They frequently appear in one area, only to disappear and reappear in other areas.

Attacks of different severity may come and go in hours or even days. The causes of transient attacks are often unknown, and the lesions may never recur. When the attacks last a few hours or days, the probability is that the attack will subside of its own accord. While that may be the case, the patient nevertheless needs relief which can be obtained via Benadryl, Atarax, ACTH and/or Prednisilone.

The origin of hives is probably internal resulting from agents in the blood and carried to the skin by the bloodstream. Urticaria lesions occur in the top layer of the skin. Angioedema, a more severe swelling, occurs in the deeper skin layers. The latter usually affects the lips, eyelids, tongue, face and genitals. Hives may be generalized. Both may appear simultaneously. Since there is no way to know whether an acute case is the beginning of a chronic case, a good patient history is essential. The most important factors are drugs, focus of infection, and food.

Physical causes such as heat or cold can be suspected if the lesions follow soon after exposure to sudden cold weather, swimming in cold (or warm) water, hot weather and water. To test for temperature sensitivity, apply an ice cube or test tube of ice water against the underside of the forearm for five or ten minutes. This produces skin wheals which are diagnostic.

A history of drug ingestion, especially aspirin, Phenopthalein (found especially in laxatives, or antibiotic drugs especially Penicillin) may be significant. Location of infection in the bladder, vagina, prostate and other areas may be of significance. My experience, though, indicates the most important focus of infection is an abscessed tooth. An examination of the mouth may show a dark tooth which may be free of all discomfort, but it may be a dead tooth. Point: all dead teeth have root infections. Elimination of this infection may well yield a clinical cure within days.

The toxins involved with an acute upper respiratory infection may also cause hives. This type of case is self-limited, but treatment for the symptoms is necessary.

In the early stage of a first occurrence of hives, the routine use of steroids suffices as a rule. If the hives return after medication is stopped, the causes suggested by the history need investigation. Hives lasting over two months are chronic and require a thorough examination. If drugs and chronic infections are first eliminated as possibilities, then food allergies ARE THE OFFENDERS IN MOST CASES.

The patient should begin an elimination diet as discussed in the chapter on food, then begin challenge feedings. Each case of hives due to food allergy must be investigated carefully because, while similar in symptoms, patients vary in food sensitivities. The general rule is that patients have food allergies in no particular pattern, and they may be allergic to one or many foods.

Three examples are cited here regarding hives lasting three months, three years, and ten years, respectively. The patient who had hives for three months was allergic to pork, black pepper, potato, and chocolate. The patient who had hives for three years was allergic to beef, black pepper, orange, sugar, peanut, onion, oat, fish, soybean, lettuce, celery cinnamon, lemon, food coloring, and shrimp. The patient who had suffered from hives for ten years was sensitive to chicken, string beans, green pepper, garlic, and vanilla. These cases are typical of patients with food allergy affecting any system of the body. Again, as far as food allergies are concerned, the only important foods are those to which the patient is allergic. Other causes may involve inhalants, emotional factors, parasitic infections, or contactants (though such cases are rare).

Patients with hives should also be investigated carefully for other allergic signs involving other body systems including respiratory, CNS, and gastrointestinal. Information concerning other body systems should be routinely included within the patient history. Although patients may seek medical help primarily for skin ailments, often there are allergies of other systems which may be of importance. A thorough history is important because patients often do not mention other symptoms because they (the patients themselves) don't consider them related to allergies!

Rachel Tyson, a 28-year-old college instructor in history at the University of Texas at Austin, came to me for treatment of chronic hives. She was also being treated at the time by a gastroenterologist for chronic recurrent duodenal ulceration and multiple gastrointestinal symptoms. And, if two doctors weren't enough, she was also seeing a third: an Eye, Nose and Throat specialist for "sinus" trouble! I hospitalized Rachel for therapeutic fasting (against her wishes!). Rachel's symptoms in all three body systems ceased once ten foods were eliminated from her diet!

Although most cases involving urticaria or angioedema can be treated successfully, there are always the few who resist every diagnostic approach. The most baffling are those involving intermittent attacks spaced weeks or even months apart. Mark Schaefer was such a patient. Mark was a 38-year-old restaurant chain owner with chronic hives of a year's duration, diagnosed by another doctor before coming to see me as "an emotional case." This conclusion had been reached by other doctors as a result of assuming that such a young man who was obviously very successful owning various businesses must be stressed to the limit. However, when I examined Mark, I found nothing of significance to indicate this or any other kind of "emotional conclusion." A diet of a few foods never or rarely eaten was ordered. He cleared in four days! But this is not the end of the story. He then broke the diet by eating one food at a time, four times a day. On the seventh day he reacted with hives within one hour after drinking tea! Mark habitually drank tea four times a day, but, off this element, he remained cured. At that point, the choice was Mark's.

Another man, 40-year-old "Willy" Simmons of Lubbock, Texas, was a water purifier installer who had widespread hives of six months duration. Upon examination, I found no foci of infection. Mr, Simmons was placed on a diet of few foods and spring water. He cleared in four days! However, all foods upon challenge failed to produce hives. The spring water was discontinued. After a few glasses of city water, his hives recurred!

Real conclusion: the cause of his allergy was the chlorine in the city water supply.

Betty Spanners, a 25-year-old music teacher in the San Antonio area, came to me with hives of two months duration. Suspecting a possible dental problem from observing a dark tooth in her mouth, I referred her to a dentist in the Port Arthur area. Dental examination and X-ray revealed an abscess had formed on her lower right molar. After proper dental care (root canal of the abscessed molar), Betty's hives left in only a few days.

# 29

## *ECZEMA*

Eczema or *atopic dermatitis* (itchy, irritating skin condition) is usually allergy related and can be eliminated with proper treatment. In infants, the lesions tend to be red, swollen areas that ooze. In older children and adults, the lesions are more often associated with a thickening of the skin. Typically, eczema affects skin folds and skin around joints. Redness and some oozing may exist chronically or at intervals, and all types of eczema itch.

This malady occurs more frequently in infants and young children than in older children and adults. When it occurs in young children, automatic remissions may happen followed by asthma and nasal allergy. Eczema also is worse in the winter and during seasonal changes.

Eczema is generally accompanied by nasal or bronchial allergy of varying intensity. While a child may show no signs of nasal or bronchial allergy in infancy, microscopic analysis of nasal secretions show large numbers of eosinophiles (blood elements that accompany allergies). That means a remission in the very young followed by nasal or bronchial symptoms is really an exaggeration of existing mild of negligible symptoms rather than an entirely new condition.

Food is traditionally considered the culprit behind eczema in infants and young children while inhalants are often blamed in older children and adults. However, my medical experience indicates that inhalants may play a role in older age groups, but food is still the major factor in all eczema in all age groups.

Traditional allergists do not recognize the importance of food as a triggering device in large part because of the diagnostic errors they make in food allergy investigations. The task of proper diagnosis is not difficult when evaluating infants. Relatively few foods are involved and one of only two foods may account for the eczema. The situation becomes dramatically complicated in other age groups. In older children and adults, multiple foods are apt to be involved. These cases tend to be misdiagnosed by traditional allergists due to the inefficient use of diets, marked inaccuracy of patient histories, and inaccuracy of traditional scratch and intradermal tests for food allergies.

The use of a diet involving a limited number of foods, as discussed in the chapter on food allergies, can bring about marked clinical improvement. Challenge feedings produce eczema flareups which provide accurate evaluation of the food allergies.

However, each case is different, and it is impossible to predict beforehand which foods are involved. In 14 eczema cases that I administered in the early '80's (ranging in ages from ten to sixty), there was no consistency in the number and variety of foods causing eczema! All of the following 14 patients recovered from the malady as well as their respiratory allergies when the offending foods or chemical items were removed from their respective diets:

Case 1.    Chocolate, orange.

Case 2.    Milk, house dust.

Case 3.    Aspirin.

Case 4.    Shellfish, black pepper, red pepper, coffee, mustard, malt, oat, vanilla, egg, chocolate, sugar, Brew's yeast, lettuce, corn.

Case 5.    Chemicals in food.

Case 6.    Milk, red pepper, tomato, peanut, caramel.

Case 7.    Milk, corn, cinnamon, red pepper, onion, malt, mustard, potato.

Case 8.    Beef, coffee, spices, peanut, tea, lemon, caramel.

Case 9.    House dust mites, shrimp.

Case 10.   Chocolate, shellfish, milk, tomato.

Case 11.   Milk, egg, beef, pork, coffee, black pepper, onion, malt, caramel, cottonseed oil.

Case 12.   Spices, orange, caramel.

Case 13.   Beef.

Case 14.   Milk, egg, coffee, corn, food color, caramel, soybean.

These patients had eczema which varied from mild to severe, but the severity of the cases did not correlate with the number of allergens involved. Some of the most severe cases had few sensitivities.

The above case examples illustrate the fact that history and statistical importance of food cannot be depended upon for diagnosis! These numbers of foods involved indicate the difficulty of food diagnosis without rigid dietary controls, preferably by therapeutic fasting in a controlled atmosphere. Most of those 14 cases were diagnosed using therapeutic fasting followed by challenge feeding.

Inhalants can be associated with food in causing eczema, but inhalants are seldom the only cause. House dust mites and animal dander may be perennial factors. Seasonal flareups may be specifically due to pollens. On several occasions I have induced eczema flareups while doing provocative skin testing with house dust mites. Molds do not fit into this accidental situation. If inhalants used in provocative skin testing do not cause visible or subjective reactions (itching), inhalants are ruled out as a cause of eczema.

What has been written thus far covers the clinical side of allergy. It is with every intention to stress that allergy covers many fields and not just asthma and nasal allergy, commonly called hay fever. Every system of the body may be affected, thus causing symptoms which are too frequently ignored by traditional approaches. As a result, millions needlessly suffer from headaches', depression, fatigue, arthritis, hyper- and hypoactivity, simply wandering about through the course of their everyday lives without any hope of receiving relief. By the use of provocative nasal tests, oral food, and chemical tests the correct diagnoses can indeed be made.

Immunity can be produced against the vast majority of allergens causing the symptomatology of allergenic patients. After extensive treatment by injection or elimination of the allergens causing the patient's reactions, a cure or near cure can be obtained within three to five months. If this is not accomplished, then SURELY ANY FURTHER TREATMENT IS DOOMED! At that time, a reevaluation of the case is necessary to find a missing link or links in the case under question. If testing proceeded by the methods advocated, the patient is safe and, in time, the answer to the problem will be found.

When the patient has been well for a period of time, there may be a flareup of symptoms that may only need symptomatic relief. If such therapy adequately controls the return of symptoms, that is well and good. But, if a week or two of relief and the elimination of medication is followed by a return of the symptoms, it may be necessary to reevaluate the case in question. By use of provocative retesting, a specified diagnosis can be made and the causative factors further isolated and ultimately eliminated.

Two case studies illustrate the importance and reliability of the technique of provocative tests. Wilma Barnett, a 42-year-old life insurance salesperson with New York Life, had been completely well for over two years when she developed severe nasal allergy manifested by sneezing and congestion of two months duration. Provocative tests for pollens and molds proved negative. Nasal tests for insects gave marked reactions to spiders and crickets. Repeat tests the following day were also positive. The history revealed that the area in which Wilma lived had an unusual number of crickets and spiders that particular past spring due to the excessively dry climate. To confirm this diagnosis, ophthalmic tests were done which showed positive. Specific therapy yielded complete relief within three months.

Jo Ann Reynolds, a 70-year-old retired dental office manager for a large practice in Houston, had chronic bronchial asthma. She was hospitalized in a controlled environment and placed on a regimen of therapeutic fasting with symptomatic therapy. Within four days she was clear of symptoms. Food challenges indicated reactions to multiple foods. She was discharged on a strict diet and was cured of asthma. However, within six months she began to have mild symptoms of the asthma reappear. Previously, Jo Ann showed negative to all inhalants. She was again placed on a diet for food elimination with only help over the phone from my office. Provocative tests for molds was again done and showed negative. A provocative skin test to house dust mites produced marked asthma. Within three months of therapy to house dust mites complete relief was obtained.

This point needs to be hammered home. NOT INFRE-QUENTLY, THE VERY BEST OF CLINICAL RESULTS CAN BE INTERRUPTED BY THE DEVELOPMENT OF NEW SEN-SITIVITIES! This is not overly worrisome, but it is a problem that has to be dealt with head-on. And we can solve these complicated problems as long as dependable provocative testing is used to uncover these mysteries.

# 30

## *A GENERAL DISCUSSION*

Usual methods of allergy investigation have been shown to be based upon skin tests which have a low diagnostic efficiency. By the use of provocative nasal tests with dried powder, the diagnostic efficiency is raised to a 90 per cent level or better. This is a far contrast of over 60 percentage points better than is registered by intracutaneous tests! The scratch test has a fairly high percentage of efficiency but, unfortunately, is too often of negative value.

In the past year or two there have been several studies showing the intracutaneous test as having a fairly high diagnostic value as proved by provocative nasal tests. The flaw in the results of these various studies is that solutions of extracts were used in such tests, NOT DRIED POWDER OF INHALANT ANTIGENS! The solutions were hypertonic, and in most cases such solutions cause mild local reactions regardless of what is used! Only through the use of powdered antigens of house dust, molds, pollens, or insects can actual symptoms show positive. Anything less is unreliable.

Again, it is emphasized that allergy covers all systems of the human body which cause illnesses of a vague nature which are generally treated symptomatically under various names and without help but at great expense of time and money. The fact is, every system of the body may be involved in any specific allergy.

The nose and throat may be involved with resultant surgical intervention BUT WITHOUT RELIEF. This mythical patient might well be cured if the allergy is recognized and one or more foods or inhalants are removed after being recognized as culprits. The use of a microscope to examine nasal secretions is a simple, harmless method to determine if allergy truly exists. If eosinophiles predominant, an allergy is present, and, if neutrophiles and bacteria are found, this indicates the presence of infection. Or, per chance, the patient with chronic headaches can easily be misdiagnosed and spend many worthless hours of examination and expense, use of medication that doesn't work and perhaps psychological treatment when a few or even just one food can be eliminated from the diet which might lead to an instant cure.

Think of the many cases of chronic fatigue and depression which are truly based upon allergy, perhaps due to a single food or preservative. The gastrointestinal tract sufferer can experience recurrent and persistent ulcers, gas, bloating, and general discomfort without ever knowing that the problem really resides within the scope of allergy WHICH WASN'T EVEN CONSIDERED IN THE DIFFERENTIAL DIAGNOSIS! Arthritis is frequently due to food allergy which is not considered, but the erroneous use of drugs is continuously used with little real relief for long periods of time! Give me a break! These cases are far too commonly misdiagnosed and treated with needless medication.

All these many conditions may well be due to allergy improperly diagnosed by doctors of multiple specializations. People go for years with such maladies and learn to live with them, but such living cannot possibly give them the pleasure they could have if properly diagnosed. Perhaps the worst offenders of all are allergists who depend in great part tests and blood work for any final diagnosis.

EVERY PATIENT WITH A CHRONIC CONDITION WHO DOES NOT RESPOND TO GENERAL THERAPY MIGHT WELL HAVE AN ALLERGIC EVALUATION BASED UPON PROVOCATIVE TESTS, ONLY! Such an evaluation done properly takes, at most, one to two, perhaps three weeks. Then, if allergic therapy is necessary, the patient should be well in three to five months.

Again, let's go back to the drawing board and see exactly what I'm talking about concerning provocative tests, and in no uncertain terms. Bobby Wise, a 14-year-old highly tauted junior chess champion and high school freshman in the Houston area, came to me with chronic asthma in the late '70's. He was found to be allergic to house dust for which he underwent one year of treatment with another doctor near my office in Port Arthur with no improvement. Bobby's original doctor in the Houston area had already run skin tests for house dust with no results, yet had continued to see Bobby for two years. Bobby was tested using nasal provocative methods with powdered antigens of inhalants. One mold was found to cause a severe allergic reaction, namely, Stemphillium Botrytis. The test was repeated and again asthma resulted within five minutes. With this one mold, specific therapy was initiated and Bobby was cured within three months. Two years later, Bobby's mother suggested stopping therapy since her child had been well for two years. A provocative nasal test with Stemphillium Botrytis was administered in powdered form and once again asthma occurred within a five minute period. This proved that Bobby had been completely immunized but not desensitized. I explained to the mother that if treatment stopped the immunity would gradually be lost in six to twelve months and as a result the asthmatic state would return. Fortunately, for Bobby, she listened. Treatment was continued, and one year later he failed to react to a provocative nasal test. This proved that he was no longer sensitive to that specific mold and therefore was cured. It was then explained that new sensitivities might occur and even resensitization was a possibility, though remote. Treatment was stopped, and two years later Bobby was still free of asthma.

Martina Fordham, a 65-year-old retired TV news anchorperson with CBS in New Orleans, at that time living in the Port Arthur area, had localized discomfort in the lower mid chest for a few months. She had gone to a reputable clinic and received evaluation by an internist followed by a gastrointestinal specialist, as well as a cardiologist. Twenty X-rays were taken of the chest, heart, and the gastrointestinal tract. Results proved negative. My spot diagnosis was chronic spasm of the pyloris, which is a muscular band at the end of the stomach. Further questioning revealed a history of daily headaches of 30 years duration for which she took six to eight aspirin tablets daily. Chronic bloating and moderate gastrointestinal discomfort had been present for years. There was also a mild nasal congestion, post nasal drip, and occasional sneezing in the morning. Previous examinations over the years from other doctors proved negative, and Martina's condition had been assumed to be emotional. This directly pointed to a case of both nasal, CNS, an gastrointestinal allergy. She was obviously quite overweight and had let herself go since retiring from the TV cameras some ten years before. Tests for inhalants proved negative.. An allergy diet was ordered which contained several foods rarely or never eaten. After four full days at home on this diet, she reported 100 per cent clearance of all symptoms. She then broke the diet one food at a time on a schedule of every three or four hours. This type of challenge took two weeks to complete, and about 30 foods and condiments were involved Martina took a full two months, however, for accurate evaluation which gave adequate time to test about 60 foods and dozens more condiments. Ten foods and condiments we're targeted to which she registered positive. She had also lost 40 pounds during the testing period, much to her delight. The financial cost to Martina before coming to see me in Port Arthur was almost $2,500, which over the years had been paid for nothing. Today, she is well and getting immunization therapy for her food allergies with very favorable results.

Margie Williams, a 50-year-old waitress in the Houston area, came to my office with chronic gastrointestinal symptoms, chronic frequent headaches and moderate diarrhea. She had six abdominal operations for intestinal ulcers in the past. At each surgery, a segment of bowl was removed which contained the ulcer. Hospitalization for a therapeutic fast was ordered. After a four-day fast, there was a remission of all symptoms. She had reacted positively to seven foods, the worst reaction being to coffee which she drank five to seven times a day. I had stayed in touch with her over the years, and up to the time I left Port Arthur, there had been no recurrence of such ulcers while maintaining her diet.

Lucy Stillman, a 60-year-old housewife, came to me with chronic bronchial asthma of a number of years duration. On a limited diet of a few foods never or rarely eaten, she was cleared of all asthma in five days. She reacted to one food element, namely, food color. Diet grape Shasta provided this food color. One element causing asthma is not rare, though I have found that the average case is allergic to nine foods or additives. Diet grape Shasta contains red #2, blue #1, and yellow #5. This drink is used exclusively for any test involving food coloring. With this simple procedure, Lucy was cured.

Evelyn Ankers of Port Arthur, a 65-year-old housewife, came to my office complaining of chronic diarrhea and gastrointestinal symptoms of two years duration, but progressively worse the past six months. This patient was a former employee of mine, serving as a laboratory technician for a number of years. She had been diagnosed by a specialist in the area and treated for ulcerative colitis with little relief. I obviously asked her straight way why she hadn't come to me sooner, and she yelled that I was an allergist! I practically screamed right back at her and reminded this wonderful lady of her nasal allergy associated with headaches which I bad successfully treated years before. I then brought up her rheumatoid arthritis during the same meeting which had been of an allergic nature and cured by omitting one food, namely, tomato. I wanted to know why she had not considered allergy when her intestinal problem had developed. She replied that she thought of this but the specialist treating her supposed "ulcerative colitis" and paid no mind to the suggestion. I put her on a limited diet and 12 days later she called to report a complete cure! One food (and one that had not been a cause from years before), milk, had caused all her trouble. 1 explained that there was a digestive enzyme called lactase which converted the lactose in milk to other ingredients. If this enzyme was missing, the undigested lactose would cause digestive disturbances INCLUDING DIARRHEA. Buttermilk was ordered as a trial. If no symptoms developed from buttermilk, it would show that an allergy was not present, but a lactose intolerance was the root problem. She drank buttermilk daily for five days and was completely free of any abnormal symptoms. milk was not the cause but rather a lactose intolerance. Ten to twenty per cent of the population have this problem, and now regular milk is on the market containing the lactase enzyme and making regular milk within toleration limits. This case example was a chance visit by an old friend had not seen in years.

Tommy Thorpe, a six-year-old first-grader in the Houston area, came to my office with chronic bronchial asthma associated with marked hyperactivity. This was manifested by constant bodily movement and jumping up and down. He was hospitalized for a therapeutic fast and cleared completely of asthma and hyperactivity within three days. All foods and condiments proved negative with the exception of peanuts.,,, Within 30 minutes of eating peanuts Tommy became hyperactive and asthma developed. A laxative dose of Milk of Magnesia cleared all his symptoms within two hours. He regularly ate peanut butter twice daily at school, then in the evening at home. Peanut was the culprit, and the Thorpe family rejoiced at so simple a cure to such a potentially devastating problem.

Mark Waylons, a ten-year-old fifth-grade boy in the Port Arthur area, came to see me with chronic asthma and showed negative on testing with all inhalants to house dust, mites, pollens, and molds. He was then hospitalized for a therapeutic fast and cleared in three days. All foods proved negative. He was discharged completely well but within two days returned to his former asthmatic state. This was evidence of what? You guessed it. Chemicals in the air, namely, $SO_2$, so prevalent in the Port Arthur area of Texas. Mark was then isolated to his room equipped with an air purifier mediated by charcoal and purifil filters. A window air conditioner was used for comfort. Such a unit, as I have discussed previously, recycles used air and, therefore, does not introduce contaminated air from the outside. He was completely well within two days. The air purifier was turned off but restarted when Mark returned home for the night. As long as the air purifier was used continuously for six to ten hours at night, Mark was free of asthma. Rather than use an air purifier with its relative inconvenience, the Waylons family eventually moved away from the area where Mark remained completely well. But when the family made a trip back to Port Arthur for a visit with relatives, Mark returned to an asthmatic state within two days. He quickly recovered when a return home was made away from the Port Arthur area. A side note: whenever the Waylons family traveled to Houston, Mark's symptoms got worse sooner than at Port Arthur.

These case studies seem simple to read, as they are certainly simple to understand. Yet many readers probably find it difficult to fully comprehend how devastating these problems are to those who suffer from these menaces WITH NO APPARENT HOPE. That's why over fifty years of medical experience in the field of allergy has been condensed into this work, to put SIMPLICITY into the hands of those who need it: THE PATIENTS.

# 31

## *ALLERGY AND SPECIFIC THERAPY*

The best treatment for any case of allergy is simply removal of the cause. If a family cat is the cause of a chronic allergy, it is obviously better to remove the cat than subject the sufferer to extensive specific treatment. If this is not possible, specific therapy can be administered with perfect or near perfect results. Case in point: Mary Seims, a 70-year-old widow with moderate asthma, was examined in my office in Port Arthur in the early '80's and determined to be allergic to cat dander. This was the entire cause of her problem. She then stated that when she awakened in the morning her cat would be sleeping in the bed close to her face, causing her to wheeze heavily in the early morning hours. She was told to get rid of the cat. The patient left the office and never returned. Perhaps that was a mistake on my part. If an error in judgment was made, it was simply this: she could have kept the cat and started specific therapy for cat dander. At least the choice could have been hers. Sorry, Mary.

The idea of therapy is to develop an immunity in the affected patient. If mites, molds, pollens, or animal dander are etiological factors, an extract of these factors is made and diluted to tolerance. If a mold extract is made, for example, and injected into the subcutaneous tissue of the patient, a reaction will definitely occur. If the injected material is too strong in its dilution, it will produce a local swelling within minutes. If overly strong, if may as well produce an attack of clinical allergy, such as sneezing or wheezing within 30 minutes, or so. To stop such a reaction, an injection of epinephrin suffices in the great majority of cases. If the reaction is mild or moderate, it will dissipate within an hour or less without medication. An extremely large overdose could produce a dangerous reaction, but such a situation is of rare occurrence.

Each injection stimulates the body to form antibodies which in time brings about a clinical cure. Such treatment injections are given at intervals. As an example, such treatments can be given as much as twice weekly for a month, then once weekly for months, then once every two weeks for three months, then once monthly. Different antigens or allergens can be mixed and given in one injection. If a local reaction occurs, as typified by a local swelling at the injection site and lasting several hours or more, reduce the next dose. If no local reaction occurs, gradually increase the subsequent doses. The top dose should leave a local swelling lasting about 12 hours with no real tenderness. Each injection stimulates the formation of antibodies which in time leads to a cure or near cure within three to five months. If this does not occur, the patient should be retested with the hope of finding the missing etiological factor. A search might implicate a new food, an inhalant, or some food preservative. For example, in a national survey published in the New England Journal of Medicine in the late '70's, 200 patients were tested with sodium nitrite. Result? Fourteen per cent reacted with clinical symptoms. This chemical food additive is found in bacon, ham, and sausage. If a patient with asthma, as summarized above, still ate the foods containing sodium nitrite, symptoms would certainly continue. Rechecking a patient and finding sodium nitrite as a missing link could well solve the problem.

Treatment should continue for two or more years. Provocative nasal tests with the specific inhalants used in treatment, if negative, would denote a cure. If reactions occurred to the inhalants, treatment should be continued until such tests prove negative. A negative reaction means a loss of sensitivity which needs to be the case if a true cure has been achieved. This discussion, then, on specific treatment, concerns inhalants such as house dust, mites, molds, pollens, animal dander, and insects. All allergists, medical doctors, and those connected to medicine accept the parameter stated within this paragraph.

However, foods and chemicals are another matter! Injections to produce immunity are not universally accepted. At least in my 50 years in the field of allergy practice I have yet to see food injection therapy used to promote or produce an immunity as is found with inhalants.

One specific group in the field of allergy uses what is *called neutralizing food injections,* but this method is not accepted by other major allergy societies. Since a specific food is generally accepted as causing an allergy, it is only reasonable to assume that injecting food extracts into a human will yield a specific formation of antibodies to combat a food allergy! BUT, FOR SOME REASON, SPECIFIC THERAPY FOR FOOD ALLERGY HAS NEVER BEEN USED TO ANY EXTENT.

# 32

## *THE MICROSCOPE IN THE ALLERGY OFFICE*

In 1935, 1 started private practice, specializing in the combination of pediatrics and allergy. The previous year I had purchased a book on allergy by Dr. French Hansel who was a specialist of some note at the time in the field of Ear, Nose, and Throat. Dr. Hansel was a true pioneer and the pathfinder of allergy within his discipline. His book was superb and became my bible. Later, we met, and that meeting turned into a lifelong friendship. He studied cytology (structure of cells) as it related to nasal secretions. By the use of a microscope, these secretions could be identified as containing bacteria, neutrophiles, or eosinophiles. If neutrophiles and bacteria predominated in the patient, then infection was present. A cure in several days would occur with the proper choice of antibiotics. If eosinophiles predominated, this indicated the presence of an allergy. So, the use of a microscope to differentiate between allergy and infection or a combination of the two was paramount in his work.

As a result of Dr. Hansel's work, Ear, Nose, and Throat specialists woke up to the predominant place allergy played in that particular specialty. This was followed by the establishment of a new specialty of allergy within the already established division of Ear, Nose, and Throat. This recognition was followed by a tremendous drop in the rate of surgical intervention! That is to say, surgery was now not an answer to allergy.

To identify various components of nasal or bronchial secretions, a good stain is necessary. The best and most useful is Dr. Hansel's stain. The whole procedure ran be finished in five minutes or less. Although deceased many years now, Dr. Hansel's stain is still available. While in active practice, I used a pint of this stain every month. On one occasion I jokingly accused Dr. Hansel of making a fortune from the sale of his stain. I remembering saying that if he sold a pint to 1,000 doctors or laboratories each month to detect allergy, he would be able to retire in a short period of time. He looked at me, then said, "Do you think everyone is like you? Most sales amount to one ounce a year!" The following point is now offered to demonstrate the overall acceptance then (circa '35) and to show you, the reader, that things haven't changed much since Lou Gehrig retired from the Yankees. Dr. Hansel then said that he had sent out brochures to over 500 pediatricians in the south, explaining the technique, its use, and the need of such a stain for the proper identification of eosinophiles and its relationship to allergy. Upon request, he offered to send these physicians an ounce bottle of the stain and directions for its use: FREE OF CHARGE. He then asked me to guess how many responses he received. I guessed wrong. Way wrong. THE ANSWER WAS ZERO. Not one.

Today, nearly 60 years later, the same situation exists,

Ignorance is as divine authority. Even to this day, I still use this stain when I feel a need to differentiate between nasal and bronchial secretions. It answers the question, "Is it allergy or infection or a combination of the two?"

# 33

## *ALLERGY IN THE ARMY*

In 1942, I entered the U. S. Army as a medical officer. Stationed at a hospital in Oklahoma, I worked where thousands of soldiers trained. My work dealt mostly with out-patients, taking care of civilians connected to the war effort. Since I was a qualified allergist, any allergy patients admitted to the hospital came under my domain.

Allergy was somewhat of a frustration, as the general attitude among doctors was that allergy was due to "psychological factors"! To make things worse, even medical officers of high rank made periodical visits of inspection, and each one down to the last would brush off allergy as due to psychological factors.

Asthma patients in training did well enough at rest, but during the rigors of field service with concomitant exercise and exposure to weather conditions these patients had real difficulty, a lot of the time ending up in the hospital. With rest, even atmospheric temperatures, and freedom of inhalants, they did fairly well. These were not *cry babies,* but, for the most part, patients who suffered from true allergies. However, the diagnosis that was most demanded by higher authority was *psychoneurosis*. Remember, before a patient could be discharged from the U. S. Army with asthma (General Discharge under medical conditions), he had to "come through" the allergy department. The asthmatic soldiers were very upset at time of separation when they learned that the diagnosis was stamped, *psychoneurosis*. Any soldier so labelled soon realized that upon returning home, a prospective employer would naturally check the reason for early discharge and find a "mental condition" as the cause of early separation. Quite clearly, the potential employer would lose interest in the possible hire, and the poor soldier's life was not very promising with such a black spot on his service record. Sorry, but that was how it was, like it or not.

On two occasions, I diagnosed soldiers with asthma, having etiological factors of house dust allergy. At this time, I had a superior house dust which would bring on an attack of asthma if used in a concentrated form of overdose. I called in a number of medical officers to act as witnesses. By giving overdoses of this potent dust extract, the patients went into attacks of real asthma. Adrenalin caused the attacks to subside. One of the medical officers signed papers attesting to the asthmatic reactions brought on with the overdoses of house dust. Another officer left with a smirk on his face as he pointed to his own head and slammed the door on the way out. Within minutes, one of the asthmatics had a severe recurrence and his skin began to break out with hives. I asked the nurse to call the doubting officer, but he just told her to write it down. Hot to the gills, I personally got this officer on the phone and demanded he return as a witness. He did return, looked at the hives in disbelief, and signed the papers which guaranteed a discharge under the conditions of bronchial asthma.

Please understand that this particular medical officer was a top-grade internist. He was not just some doctor assigned to the "outpost country of Oklahoma. " The very same thing goes on today among very good doctors. But, I must say, there has been improvement in attitudes over the years. Shortly after this incident, I talked to the colonel who was also chief of the medical service. I stressed the general attitude that medical officers had concerning allergy and volunteered to hold a special clinic to demonstrate specific causes of allergies due to inhalant sensitivity. During this particular time, molds were not in clinical use, but some investigating was proceeding in this field. An allergist from Chicago had published an article on several molds he had isolated from the air. He had responded to a pleading letter and sent to me five small vials containing I gm each of the five molds. I checked several patients with asthma admitted to the hospital in Oklahoma who had cleared due to "clean air. " Provocative nasal tests were done and four of the patients reacted with asthma to a specific mold. The fifth reacted with asthma to a lyophilized potent house dust powder. It was these five asthmatics who were presented to the medical officers present at the weekly medical seminar.

The doctors present were asked to examine these five soldiers to be sure the soldiers had no evidence of asthma. NO ONE GOT UP TO CHECK THE SOLDIERS. The chief of medicine then volunteered to examine them and within a few minutes announced to all present that the soldiers were clear of any signs of asthma. The nasal provocative tests then proceeded using the four molds and the lyophilized house dust powder. Five minutes later I invited the medical officers to renew the examinations and, again, A TOTAL NEGATIVE RESPONSE OCCURRED. No one was willing to offer any examination. Again, the chief of medicine volunteered. As he examined each asthmatic, he uttered such words as amazing, unbelievable, and astounding! It was like an explosion had taken place when this chief of medicine faced those present and announced that each soldier had responded with definite asthma! To my surprise, the room of medical officers applauded! FROM THAT POINT ON, ALLERGY IN THE U. S. ARMY MISLABELLED AS PSYCHONEUROSIS WAS DEAD!

Another case of interest concerns the wife of an Army man whom I saw as an outpatient. Susan Benish complained of abdominal discomfort associated with cramps and gas, which occurred frequently. On occasional days, Susan seemed well enough. She had been diagnosed as having gall bladder disease and surgery was advised. In every case of abdominal disturbance, allergy should be suspected. If there is an associated nasal congestion or post nasal drip, regardless of how mild, symptoms of allergy of the gastrointestinal system is almost a sure bet. Susan was put on a diet of only a few foods rarely or infrequently eaten. This was done for four days, after which she cleared of all symptoms. The diet was broken one food at a time, several times a day. She had a typical and moderate reaction to eggs. Relief followed in a matter of hours after a dose of Milk of Magnesia. Susan remained well on a diet of egg elimination.

Not the end of the story! A week or so later, Susan called, complaining that she had an attack of abdominal discomfort. She insisted she had not eaten any eggs or any food contaminated with egg products. A close history revealed that she had eaten ice cream without trouble, but, upon repeating the ice cream test the next day, trouble followed. The two ice creams were analyzed as to contents. One of the two was made without eggs, the other with eggs. The one with the eggs was the culprit. Detective work is often involved which the patient can readily do with initial guidance. TRUST ME ON THIS ONE: A GOOD PERCENTAGE OF TODAY'S DOCTORS WOULD IGNORE THE IMPORT OF SUSAN'S STORY.

Fifty years have passed since my U. S. Army days. Yet with this lapse of time, a sizable segment of medical people still connect allergy with emotions! There is no doubt that emotions play a prominent role in medicine, BUT IT HAS NO SPECIFIC ETIOLOGICAL ROLE IN ALLERGY. Of course, emotional upsets can aggravate allergic conditions just as it will aggravate many other diseases. But giving a patient a new personality will not clear a case of asthma which has an etiology due to milk or eggs!

I left the U. S. Army in 1945, at which time I returned to private practice. About 1948 or so, if memory serves correctly, I attended an allergy meeting. The guest speaker was an allergist who was considered an expert on molds, which was rather new at the time but was becoming prominent in clinical allergy practice. At the end of this talk, I discussed his paper and agreed that molds were important. However, I questioned the accuracy of the etiological tests being used. The speaker reacted a little antagonistically and said, "If you do not believe in mold allergy, just take a plate of molds and let an allergic patient sniff the plate!" I snapped my fingers, sat down, and said to myself, "Never let me forget this and keep me from falling into the same trap as did the medical officers I briefed in Oklahoma! Wake up and think!"

Upon returning home from the seminar, I converted all my skin tests to powdered antigens and started routine provocative nasal tests. Astounding results followed, and a new life of promise opened for me and my patients for years to come.

CASE: One of the medical officers after much hesitation conferred with me about his chronic nasal symptoms, which were getting to be of some concern. Allergy was a blind object to him. I found specific inhalants as the probable cause of his trouble and suggested three months of therapy to prove ALLERGY was no figure of speech. To his great surprise he was clinically well. He was bewildered and still in some doubt as if I had some magic control. so he stopped treatment and within several weeks was well again. He was convinced and continued. In case of being shipped overseas, I left him adequate supplies.

This was the mental state that allergy faced some fifty years ago and you can well believe this state of mind still persists in far too great a segment of the medical profession.

CASE: Back in that same period of time (some fifty years ago) Joyce Overton, the wife of a medical officer had chronic asthma. Her husband was in the psychiatric department and this type of mental control was practiced on this poor woman. No results. Since I ran the allergy section he very reluctantly asked for possible help. I was out within days, so after a thorough exam I was optimistic and planned out a whole routine of therapy. After I left I would have bet dollars to dirt that my planning, medication and instructions were dumped with no regrets.

It must be admitted that allergy therapy and testing is far from perfect as generally used. This is the purpose of this book which supplies new, improved insights of proven value.

CASE: Matt Fredricks, a 20-year-old private, had chronically inflamed eyes of one year's duration. The condition had been blamed on tear duct infection. There were not any antibiotics at this period. A cytology study of the eye secretions revealed no signs of infection, but there were 4 plus eosinophiles which proved the allergic diagnosis. A local test using a tiny amount of lyophiled powder of house dust gave an immediate reaction proving an allergic factor. Treatment was not started for he was discharged.

# 34

## ODORS AND GASES IN THE AIR

Odors and gases in the air come from various sources and may well act as potential allergens. These allergens exist in every home and emanate from industrial sources to reach both inside and outside air for all to breathe. As such, allergy as a discipline is becoming more prominent due to greater industrialization and commercial development.

Gone are the days when house dust, pollens , foods and molds were the only etiological factors in general allergy. With industrial progress came gases, odors, chemicals and all affect food supply. A modern home couldn't be built without chemically infested wood and wood substitutes. All these chemical additions play a significant part in our health. Human beings have not been able to completely adapt to these foreign substances and far too frequently allergies and toxic conditions arise.

Morgan Baines, a 54-year-old plumber, came to me in the early '80's, not as a patient but, as a man searching for medical advice. He had respect for me as a doctor as in the past I had cured his wife of rheumatoid arthritis which was of an allergic nature.

This man had developed a crippling gait and would fall upon walking only a few yards. As a result, he had been forced to take early retirement. He had received no relief from medical treatment. I made a preliminary diagnosis: a possible CNS allergy. Some food or chemical was suspected as the culprit. He was admitted to St. Mary's where the air was free of outside chemicals. The hospital room was free of all plastics or any fixtures which might contaminate the air. He was placed on a therapeutic fast. After a full four days, he could walk up and down the hallway and around his room without aid and with a normal gait. This seemed an obvious case of food allergy. The diet was broken one food at a time and, to even my surprise, he failed to react to any food! After two more days, he was clinically well on a full diet. He was discharged, and after two days at home all his symptoms returned. It seemed now a sure bet that sulphur dioxide in the air was the etiological factor causing his disability. He was then isolated to his room and an air purifier installed. After four days, there was still no improvement. Chemicals were then suspected, in and about the house. A second trip to the hospital was made under the same circumstances. A full diet was again ordered, and four days later he was completely well. It now seemed that etiological factors were probably at work in the house. The patient then, on his own, consulted a neurologist with medical school affiliations in a nearby city. I concurred with his desire. The diagnosis was Parkinson's Disease. This is a disease afflicting the CNS for which no therapy exists. In time, one becomes bedridden and eventually death occurs. He had informed the neurologist about the complete cures that followed his two visits to St. Mary's Hospital. The doctor totally ignored this information. A week or so passed, after which time Morgan consulted a second neurologist who gave the same diagnosis and paid no attention to his previous St. Mary's results. At this point, the State Health Department was contacted and plans made to check the air in each room of the patient's home for chemicals in the air. Unfortunately, Morgan lost hope in this enterprise and cancelled the arrangements. The building of a new home was suggested, one with materials which were chemically free, and two books existed at that time on how to do this. However, Morgan claimed he could not afford this. At this point, I lost contact with the patient, and to this day do not know how everything turned out.

Another interesting case was that of Diane Hammond, a 75-year-old retired school teacher from Port Arthur with chronic asthma of several year's duration. Tests for inhalants proved negative. She was hospitalized for a therapeutic fast and cleared in three days. All foods showed negative. Close questioning revealed this patient had a pleasant addiction to the odor of pine oil. She used this oil for the bathroom at first and then the whole house followed. She stated that she had a most pleasant house due. to the pine oil odor. A trip to the supply room of the hospital produced a bottle of pine oil. The patient was given the pine oil to smell and in minutes she began to wheeze. A thorough cleaning of her home eliminated the pine odor and a cure followed.

# 35

# *PARENTECTOMY AND EMOTIONS*

Many years ago, an eminent allergist came up with a theory of emotional allergy or asthma occurring in children. Because of poor results otherwise, he theorized that many children with asthma had a too dependent connection with their mothers which led to asthma! A comparison to the field of criminology: a noted criminologist once stated in the early '50's that those with protruding foreheads were more apt to become criminals than those with flat foreheads! The allergist, in any event, wrote and talked about cutting the umbilical cord, separating the pair, and thus allergic relief would surely follow! Somehow, through means of which I am not entirely certain, this seemed to work and led to the formation of the Children's Asthma Hospital in Denver, Colorado. Before long, this hospital filled up with patients from all parts of the country where the children received the best of medical and nursing care. Many cases cleared up overnight, and many others were drastically improved. But enough cases remained that had been completely untouched to ask the telling question. Does this approach really work?

Patients remained for periods of one to two years before discharge. The ambulant children continued their education by going to the local schools, and the nonambulant had a regular school curriculum in the hospital itself. Many years later when mites were discovered and proved to be the specific factor in house dust, the riddle to the success even then was only partially unveiled. Since 60 to 70 per cent of asthmatics are allergic to house dust mites, it must be emphasized that mites cannot live in altitudes above 2,000 feet. Denver is the mile-high city, so enough said. It is obvious, then, that patients with asthma due to mite sensitivity would get relief upon leaving their mite-infested low-land homes and entering the promised land of the Denver Broncos.

The fresh air we breathe contains foreign matter such as gases and odors, all of which may well contain etiological allergy factors. What we eat, breathe, and smell can be isolated, however, and checked as allergy factors which might well answer the many secrets which may be etiological factors in the health of those that suffer from allergies.

# 36

## *ALLERGY AND REAL RESULTS*

Any degree of improvement is frequently considered as falling in the range of "good results. " I have already emphasized that if, after three to five months of specific therapy, a patient is not cured or near cured further treatment is of little value. It is then time to reevaluate the case and search for the missing allergen or allergens that may be perpetuating the allergic condition. On several occasions over the years, I tested patients with preservatives which were not checked previously. Sodium nitrite and sulphite proved positive in numerous cases. The patients cleared up completely as a result of eliminating foods containing the guilty chemicals.

Many years ago and before using provocative tests, my patients were judged by different criteria with many results questionable but still considered favorable. After introducing provocative tests, etiological factors were more evident and better results followed. Generally, those allergists using skin tests for diagnosis have an efficiency of only around 30 per cent against provocative nasal tests with dry powdered antigens which is about 90 per cent truly diagnostic.

Surely hospitalization for therapeutic fasts followed by food challenges is of major importance. The statistics here are enlightening. In checking 1,000 patients in this manner, 50 per cent had an allergic etiology of both foods and inhalants, 25 per cent had reactions to foods, and 25 per cent had reactions to inhalants alone.

What about the findings of other allergists? At a recent meeting of allergists in the mid west, I questioned a number of doctors concerning their findings. None agreed with mine, and all had findings which varied from A to Z. Yet, despite these differences, all seemed to be satisfied with what they were currently doing and the subsequent results. So, what's the truth about allergy? The reader will have to make up his own mind.

Moreover, a very knowledgeable and able allergist recently published the findings of a telethon in which he participated. It dealt with bronchial asthma and was sponsored by a steroid inhaler manufacturer. This allergist was amazed at how many patients under therapy were on inhalant steroids for relief. He stated that more than one allergist had 80 per cent of his patients on them! Yet, in his practice, he had only eight patients on inhaler steroids! How can this be? You tell me. What is a "clinical result"?

I have yet to meet an allergist who is not seemingly satisfied with the status quo. Only with improved diagnostic techniques can medical allergy reach a uniform level of perfection. So, what are we to believe? That's why you, the reader, have a mind. Use it.

# 37

## AN ALLERGY STORY? OR A BAD HABIT OF BREATHING?

Approximately 60 years ago, my father, Avrohm Hosen, lived in Mississippi while I was in my first year of practice in another city. A friend and classmate of mine lived and practiced in my father's town. This friend was the family doctor. He wrote and told me that my father had developed a heart problem, and he advised my father to visit me so that I could get a proper specialist for him. But, you see, there were no heart specialists at that time in his or my area. An excellent cardiologist did, however, live not far away who just happened to be the chief of cardiology at a medical school.

My father arrived at my house completely free of symptoms at that particular time, though he reported on two different occasions while walking he had suddenly developed some chest pain and had difficulty breathing. However, once rested, he felt fine and would continue his walking.

The following day he came to my office where we tested a very good extract of house dust on a few patients, just to see what skin reaction might occur to those who had no allergy symptoms. We included my father in this procedure. I had left the room and within minutes heard my father sneeze a few times. Then he called me to come quickly as he could not breathe. Realizing that we had precipitated an attack of asthma, I hurriedly administered an injection of adrenalin to relieve the asthma. Obviously, my father's "heart problem" was asthma brought on by exertion. I then recalled my teen years and thought about my father's problem in quite a different light. He would often sneeze several times when he took the family to the movies. I would ask him what was wrong and he answered that it was a little passing cold. So, this kind of allergy did indeed go back for years, but it was of minor import.

The cardiologist then examined my father. He said he was one of the healthiest men for his age he had ever seen! In spite of my message regarding allergy, the cardiologist, though, concluded that my father just had a bad habit of breathing incorrectly! He said the adrenalin shot was additional proof of freedom from any heart disorder because it did not activate any heart symptoms. Upon returning to my house, my father said, "He may be a big heart specialist, but this is not *a habit. I* have something wrong. "

The following day, my father was put through a complete allergy examination at my clinic, and only house dust was tagged as a factor. Treatment was started and within two months of therapy he was completely cured. With additional treatment, he remained well.

Many such cases exist of people who do well enough without allergy therapy, but specific therapy keeps the patients feeling young and free of fear (nerves). This term *nerves* is still in vogue for allergy patients, especially when treatment is a failure and the doctor is at a loss to explain things in any other way.

The doctor and classmate of mine who referred my father to me retired many years later and settled on the Gulf Coast. We had not seen each other for many years, so his long distance call one day was a pleasant surprise. He was having nasal problems which had reached an aggravating state. He assumed he had a case of nasal allergy. We arranged for hospitalization to investigate possible food allergy. An office examination ruled out allergy to inhalants. Cytology studies showed evidence of an allergic condition and no infection. In the hospital setting, he cleared up completely using therapeutic fasting. On the fourth day, his fast was broken one food at a time, and we determined that he was allergic to four foods.

Even he was amazed that I had found a clinical cure with just the elimination of four foods! Since he could easily find ample substitutes for those foods, he preferred not to take treatment but just eliminate them from his diet. This retired doctor was astonished to say the least and told me that he would call after a trial period. One month later he did just that and said he was cured of all symptoms. This good friend was now a believer in the relationship between allergies and the human condition.

# 38

# *HEADACHES*

Headaches are one of our most common complaints in the field of clinical medicine. It is a term frequently associated with the nervous system. Frequently the sinuses involved. Headaches as an emotional outlet may be a factor but this diagnosis is more frequently wrong than right. The sinus involvement can be easily overlooked, for minor sinus or nasal symptoms can be easily overlooked. With headaches gastrointestinal symptoms, depression, fatigue and sundry symptoms may exist. All of these involvements may well be associated. Allergy figures prominently with all these symptoms.

Sharon Reed, a 50-year-old South Texas woman, complained of frequent headaches, depression and fatigue. Many medical examinations were of no avail. The final diagnoses of several doctors spelled out NEUROSES. She came as a patient for a possible allergy which was different and spelled out possible hope.

Inhalants were negative on provocative nasal testing so she was admitted to the hospital for therapeutic fasting. After a period of four days there was a complete remission of all previous symptoms so foods were added every 3 to 4 hours. I paid my usual morning visit and found Sharon in tears of frustration. Her previous meal consisted of 1 tablespoon of plain SUGAR. Within minutes it seemed she reacted with headache, depression and fatigue. These symptoms were soon controlled following the elimination of her gastrointestinal contents. The tears were of frustration due to the thought that for years she had suffered needlessly. Two other foods reacted.

By mere chance twenty years later I was in the area where Sharon lived. By mere chance we met again. She was elated and told me she was still free of trouble.

This is not an odd story for I can duplicate this many times over.

Forty-five-year-old Donna Schneider of North Central Texas came to me for help with her chronic headaches for I had treated her husband successfully for asthma. He was so enthusiastic that he insisted that his wife's headaches might be allergy related. After a four-day fast she was clinically well. on breaking her fast Donna developed a typical headache after consuming one simple food. This brought tears of frustration to think that a food caused years of suffering when help was only a short distance away.

Any unsolved headache should be considered as due to an allergy, especially if there is an associated involvement of sinusitis or any other system of the body. This is something any patient can self-evaluate as I will later point out.

Migraine is a common household word and it is usually and wrongfully applied to any so-called sick headache. Migraine is a diagnosis escape valve which unfortunately keeps the sufferer from getting proper relief.

Migraine has specific set of symptoms which are easy to identify. A migraine patient first notices a peculiar odor with or without a flashing light occurring on one side of the head or face. This is followed by a one-sided headache of various degrees of intensity. A feeling of nausea follows, frequently followed by vomiting. Lying down in bed in a dark room gives some comfort. The headache is self-limited, lasting from hours to two or more days. This varies with the severity of the migraine attack.

Allergy has no relationship to the classical migraine. The unknown etiology originates in the brain. Excellent response with quick relief follows an injection of specific medication given early in the attack. Attacks may vary from weekly to monthly to even yearly. Aged or older patients have more infrequent attacks. If you have classical migraine, carry the injectable medication, which you can easily learn to use, with you at all times.

Check for allergy in only the so-called "migraine" headaches which are not classical. 50-year-old Margaret Scott, a patient from the Texas Panhandle with respiratory allergy which was well-controlled with specific therapy, had classical migraine. Her migraine only occurred two or three times a year and she controlled it with a self-injection of specific medication.

Later Margaret developed frequent attacks of one-sided headaches which were not classical migraine.

At this period I was investigating the chemical sodium nitrite as a possible allergen in clinical allergy. This chemical is found in all bacon, ham, and sausages. During a period of freedom of a headache several hours after a meal, Margaret was in my office. I had her sit at rest for an hour and gave her a capsule containing 40 to 50 mg. of sodium nitrite. Within minutes she developed a severe one-sided headache which cleared within minutes following an injection of adrenalin. This is a specific drug used for control of any allergy attack. Margaret was informed of the situation and as a result there were no recurrences of these headaches as long as the offending foods were eliminated.

CASE REPORT: Natalie Randall, a housewife with headaches and so-called sinus trouble was found negative to all office tests. Therapeutic fasting led to complete freedom of symptoms. On food challenge five foods were found involved, but on returning home acute symptoms recurred within a few hours.

She returned to the office and in general conversation Natalie admitted to having the sweetest smelling house in Port Arthur, Texas, my home base of clinical practice. Shortly after this interview she began to clear up obviously due to freedom from contact with the etiological factors in her home. She was ordered to smell each article in her home to help detect any item which might be a factor causing her distress. The first things which caused almost immediate trouble were Natalie's perfumed candles. Further investigation revealed four odorous cleaning fluids. old-fashioned Bon Ami which is odorless was substituted for the odorous cleaning substances and the perfumed candles took a holiday. This simple elimination of foods and odorous household objects resulted in a cure, not just relief.

CASE REPORT: Anne Lind, a 30-year-old Central Texas graduate student, suffered with headaches and nasal congestion. Medical investigations failed to give relief. History taking revealed that Anne's symptoms occurred especially at night and early in the morning. Some relief followed breakfast but great relief followed leaving her home during the day. The history pointed especially to her bedroom. The most important etiological factor in the bedroom is the pillow made of synthetic material.

Routinely I kept six new cotton pillows in the office to check such patients. With suspicious patients I loaned two pillows for one night's use. Anne used the pillows with complete relief. She returned to the office, paid for the cost of the pillows, gave thanks and prepared to leave. Anne was reminded that she still had minor symptoms which called for further study. With a flippant wave of her hand she departed, stating that with her great relief the other discharged as unfit for military duty. His discharge diagnosis was ALLERGIC CONJUNCTIVITIS.

# 39

## *SELF-HELP IN ALLERGY DIAGNOSIS*

This book spells out the story of clinical allergy. There are no mystical observations but only obvious facts. By observation and by routinely following directions, an individual can successfully investigate most etiological factors causing distress. Since a personal investigation is without any danger and can be done without any great disruption of lifestyle nothing is lost. If results are not satisfactory by all means confer with a specialist in the field of allergy.

It was emphasized in this book that 25% of allergy patients had food problems alone, 25% had problems with inhalants alone and 50% were bothered by both foods and inhalants.

With foods include chemicals (which is discussed in one chapter.) Again, don't forget that chemicals in the air such as sulphur dioxide, odors from furniture, pillows and rugs, perfumes and cleaning fluids must be included in inhalants. The major inhalants consist of house dust with its associated mites, pollens, molds and animals. Most inhalants are effectively used by provocative nasal testing to be effective, which is out of reach of the patient and must be done by the trained allergist.

The method of food investigation is spelled out, which the patient can easily follow in the home.

Many case studies are presented which fit the reader. similar observations may do wonders.

# SPECIFIC THERAPY ON FOOD ALLERGY

It seems that since the beginning of the specialty of allergy specific therapy in food allergy has been frowned upon. One group some 50-odd years ago started therapy of food allergy by a technique of so-called neutralization. This method is frowned upon by major allergy societies.

My personal investigation of this technique showed it to be of very doubtful value.

Later I used regular extracts for injection therapy for food allergy and results followed. Some years ago a chance meeting with a semiretired and older allergist brought up the subject of Allpyral extracts used as a supposedly superior method of injection therapy. This type of medication allowed for more infrequent injections with supposedly superior immunizing power. It is patented and a number of allergists believe in its superior ability to elicit better immunity.

Through the good graces of this semiretired allergist I was supplied with some food extracts which I sued with success. To make such Allpyral extracts took time and the complicated equipment was relatively expensive.

This friend died rather suddenly so I purchased his equipment from his estate and the technician came to my office to arrange the complicated equipment and to teach the necessary technique of extraction to my technician.

Good results followed the use of food extracts using this product. Three to five months of treatment made it possible for the patient to eat the forbidden foods.

After having almost completely retired and moving to another city, I ceased working with Allpyral food extraction. Then I resorted to the use of food extracts of regular manufacture and found good results. Why no one person used food injections in the past can only be conjectured. The moral that follows is that one should investigate himself any doubtful technique and not be persuaded by the dead voices of the past.

The laboratory owning this Allpyral patent allowed me to use it as long as I did not commercialize it. This laboratory also stated that when there was a demand it would make Allpyral food extracts on a commercial basis.